More Praise for *Conquering Cultural Stress*

"Through his many recommendations, including those that promote the freedom of the intuitive toddler within you, nurture a state of happiness, help manage stress, encourage healthy nutrition and physical activity habits, and engage the power of the mind through the use of positive affirmations and other techniques, Dr. Murad offers a wealth of wisdom for seekers of health and well-being in their lives and in the lives of those close to them."

—Marc J. Weigensberg, MD, Director, USC Institute for Integrative Health

"In sports, greatness is defined by the longevity of your success. Success becomes a lifestyle. Applying Dr. Murad's Inclusive Health philosophy to my professional and personal life makes it easier to shine both on and off the ice!"

—Allison Baver, three-time Olympic short track speed skater and 2010 Olympic bronze medalist

"In an era in which we are bombarded with constant demands and the need to always be 'on,' Dr. Murad's book reminds us that it is, in fact, okay to stop and turn off our phones for a while, to relax and to enjoy the small and important things in life. Not only is this essential for balance and happiness—it is also a key component to living a healthy life. As a molecular biologist, I am intrigued by the science that supports Dr. Murad's ideas —this philosophy is at the forefront of a new era in medicine."

—Anna Langerveld, PhD, President and CEO, Genemarkers, LLC

"Dr. Murad's Inclusive Health approach to managing today's cultural stress is vitally needed for these times. By following his practical wisdom and healthy lifestyle plan, you can improve the quality of your life. An essential book to help you cope with the cultural stresses you face in today's modern high-tech world."

—John Westerdahl, PhD, MPH, RD, CNS, Director, Bragg Health Institute, and host, *Health & Longevity*

"Every year or so, thousands of books are published worldwide. But only a very small fraction of these books deserve to be considered as truly transformative, iconoclastic, and consequential in terms of their overall impact on our lives. *Conquering Cultural Stress* by Dr. Murad is one such book."

—Michael P. Tabibian, MD, FAAD, Advanced Dermatology Care of Southern California, Clinical Instructor, David Geffen School of Medicine at UCLA

"Dr. Howard Murad has decoded the ultimate cause of aging—cultural stress. . . . If you read this book and apply its immense wisdom to your everyday living, you will become a healthier, happier, and more fulfilled human being."

—Jasmina Jankicevic, MD, MSc, dermatologist

"In the fast-paced world that we live in, Dr. Murad has identified the pervasive pressures that we feel daily, what he has termed 'cultural stress.' Identifying these triggers and making the effort to deal with these stressors leads to a more balanced lifestyle that reflects on our health overall and I think can improve skin health as well."

—Annie Chiu, MD, board-certified cosmetic and general dermatologist

"I have seen firsthand what an asset Dr. Murad's knowledge is to our customers. His extensive knowledge of the scientific research behind the benefits of whole foods gave our customers a deeper understanding of the effects surrounding what we eat, and his all-inclusive approach to health offered valuable insights to overall wellness and vitality that were truly empowering."

—Lisa Zollner, Marketing Team Leader, Whole Foods Market, Plaza El Segundo

"Inclusive Health has helped me feel happier! My brain feels like it functions better—with improved mental clarity and a better ability to get things done. I have more energy and am stronger—both physically and emotionally. My skin feels healthier, and others have noticed that I look better. It's basically an all-over healthier and happier way to live!"

—Rosanna Libertucci, patient

"Dr. Howard Murad is one of the most joy-filled and inspirational people I know. His approach to dealing with cultural stress gives people the tools to live healthier and happier. I recommend this book for anyone seeking new ways to transform their lives."

—Judy Brooks, Executive Producer and cohost, *Healing Quest*

"*Conquering Cultural Stress* is a profound and visionary view into longevity that provides the road map for an enriched, fulfilled journey through life. The Bellus Academy is proud to include Dr. Murad's book and philosophy in our students' experience of changing one life at a time."

—Lynelle Lynch, President, Bellus Academy

"Dr. Murad combines a wealth of medical knowledge and experience with the rare ability to see the entirety of a person, not just the patient in the room. With this he provides a unique insight into stress and well-being. In his latest book, he shares his secrets of health and stress, from the level of DNA and cells to the level of society as a whole. Mastering this knowledge will change the way the reader looks at health, stress, youth, and happiness forever."

—Andrew Breithaupt, MD

"As a family physician, I apply the lessons I learned working with Dr. Murad, such as maintaining emotional self-care, food as information, and consistent exercise to achieve dramatic improvements in the lives of my patients with chronic diseases. I am confident this book will help you transform your life as it has mine and the lives of my patients."

—Dr. Juan Ramirez, family physician

"Dr. Howard Murad has written a very useful and timely book filled with practical how-to instructions for managing the stress in our lives and minimizing the impact it has on our health, general well-being, and relationships with others. He is truly revolutionary in his approach to skin care and overall heath in recognizing that "integrative medicine"—the treatment of the mind, soul, and body—allows people find balance in their lives and effectively treat the individual diseases they are afflicted with."

—Scott Rackett, MD

"Dr. Murad's new book is a must-read that provides great insights into how to live a healthier, happier life. His wisdom about improving overall health and well-being through diet, exercise, and reducing cultural stress has provided me with both personal and professional anti-aging results for which I am very grateful."

—Susan F. Reynolds, MD, PhD, President and CEO, The Institute for Medical Leadership

"The book is a wake-up call to acknowledge the amount of stress we allow into our lives, learn what is causing it and how to lessen it, and discover how to have a happier, healthier, and longer life."

—Joan Johnson, writer and instructor, Mount St. Mary's College, Graduate Division Humanities

"Dr. Murad demonstrates compellingly the need for patients and healthcare practitioners alike to blend science, faith, and philosophy in the quest for better health, well-being, and happiness."

—Dominique M. Fradin-Read, MD, MPH

"Dr. Murad has written the optimal prescription to reverse aging and rejuvenate youthfulness. Incredible and a must-read!"

—Bernadette Anderson, MD, MPH

"Medical science has proven that a life filled with cultural stress can damage a strong physical body, bringing on illness and harmful effects. *Conquering Cultural Stress* is a masterpiece in knowledge, and with Dr. Murad's personal guidance and expertise, you will develop a greater understanding and peace of mind."

—Joel Gerson, PhD, author of *Milady's Standard Textbook for Professional Estheticians* and *Milady's Standard Fundamentals for Estheticians*

"Dr. Murad has discovered the Holy Grail of living well, feeling good, and looking great! In this easy to read book, he gives us valuable new insight for achieving happiness and overall great health through finding one's inner child and conquering 'cultural stress.' By integrating his years of clinical experience and vast scientific knowledge, he provides us simple yet key strategies of living and eating well, proving that anyone can significantly improve one's life with his ultimate healthcare secrets."

—Peter Loisides, MD

"We love Dr. Murad and his excellent advice. Anyone can learn something from his words on cultural stress—including other physicians!"

—Christina Correia, Los Angeles County Medical Association, Physician Magazine

"Dr. Murad is a visionary. He combines the mastery of science with the mystery of the human spirit to create the gift of a healthy life."

—Rocky Delgadillo, Los Angeles City Attorney (2001–2009) and CEO, Los Angeles County Medical Association

CONQUERING CULTURAL STRESS

The Ultimate Anti-Aging Secret

*3 Steps to Looking, Living,
and Feeling Better*

Howard Murad, MD

WISDOM WATERS PRESS

Wisdom Waters Press
1000 Wishire Blvd., #1500
Los Angeles, CA 90017-2457
www.wisdomwaterspress.com

Ordering Information
Quantity sales. Special discounts are available on quantity purchases by corporations, associations, and others. For details, contact the "Special Sales Department" at the address above.

Orders by US trade bookstores and wholesalers. Please contact National Book Network at (800) 462-6420 or visit www.nbnbooks.com for details.

Printed in the United States of America

Cataloging-in-Publication Data

    Murad, Howard (Professor of dermatology)
       Conquering cultural stress : the ultimate anti-aging
    secret : 3 steps to looking, living, and feeling better
    / Howard Murad, MD. -- First edition.
      pages cm
      Includes index.
      ISBN 978-1-939642059 (cloth)
      ISBN 978-1-939642066 (ebook)

      1. Aging--Prevention. 2. Aging--Psychological
    aspects. 3. Health. I. Title.
    RA776.75.M87 2015   613
    QBI14-600148

First Edition

19 18 17 16 15   10 9 8 7 6 5 4 3 2 1

Contents

Can you remember who you were, before the world
told you who you should be?

—Danielle LaPorte

PART I

RETURNING TO YOUR YOUTH IS THE PATH TO HEALTH AND HAPPINESS

My mission is to teach people how to achieve whole-body wellness, effortless weight management, and freedom from stress by returning the body's cells to more youthful qualities. And my approach is unlike those of other doctors and lifestyle experts who focus solely on diet and fitness. You're not about to read about good versus bad carbs, or why you should start measuring your blood sugar and take up running. I'm going to show you a revolutionary way to understand health and aging, as well as how to maximize your well-being. I'll reveal that by getting in touch with the unencumbered, free-spirited child you once were—whose potential was unlimited—and maintaining high levels of cellular hydration that you also had as a youth, you can age in a healthy fashion that allows you to look and feel as vibrant, happy, and young as possible. As you're about to find out, wellness, joyfulness, cellular water, and aging share a unique synergy that informs how we should live to become the best that we can be.

CHAPTER 1

How the Toddler in You Can Save Your Life

Eighty percent of health resides in the brain.

Take a moment to think about what it must have been like to be a two-year-old, because you probably don't remember those days from your own life. But you can certainly conjure something up just by looking at a toddler today or perhaps recalling the memory of your own child. Toddlers reflect the essence of youth. They are daring, creative, and inquisitive. They don't doubt or worry. "Stress" is not a word in their vocabulary. And before they were talkative little creatures, they fell down thousands of times, skinned their knees over and over again, and met more failures in their day than any adult could handle. Trial and error is their game. It's how they master scooting, crawling, then walking, and later running. And they are spontaneous in all that they do—no sense of meticulous planning for the future or aggrieved reminiscing about the past. They pretty much live in the now and are chiefly concerned only about themselves. They take things as they come and try something new every day. Their emotions are real and expressed. Whether they are screaming mad with frustration or laughing so hard that their belly aches, two-year-olds don't hide anything. They don't know how to—yet.

Then, by around the age of three they've learned to say no and to assert their wants, and they begin to fear failure. No longer are they trying to just learn from an innate sense of self and instinct. And no longer are they happy with the imperfections of their first two years. Now they want to achieve successes quickly, experience instant gratification, please their peers and parents, meet expectations, and rely less on intuition or more on the wisdom—and approval—of others. They start to be competitive and perfectionistic, and they are excellent self-critics, even if they don't know what that means. They also are acutely aware of their shortcomings and flaws. The words "I can't" begin to emerge. While they may have once possessed a primal attraction to some activity or form of learning, such as enjoying music, playing sports, watching nature, or playing with their hands in a bowl of wet paint, now they are more calculating and restrictive with their pursuits. It's as if they've lost touch with an innate spark that reflects "reckless abandon," for now they are more likely to reject their inner wisdom and instead listen to others—parents, teachers, peers. They are, in a lot of ways, adults at this juncture and highly vulnerable to the surrounding environment and culture. Much farther down this road, they may end up choosing careers that promise money but not happiness because they don't tap into their innermost unique spirit and reason for being on earth. Or they may find themselves in unhappy relationships because they don't know how to be their authentic selves and find someone who can help them do that.

Now think about your own life for a moment. Are you not spontaneous and carefree, not one who tries new endeavors frequently? Do you find yourself calculating your risks before you leap forward in an unfamiliar adventure? Do you worry about the future and harbor regrets from the past? Do you avoid your gut instinct sometimes and follow someone else's lead or advice? Do you feel down, moody, and depressed sometimes? Even though you stay tuned in to everything thanks to computers and smart phones, do you often feel isolated and disconnected from people? Do you ever hide your emotions? Do the high expectations you place on yourself as well as those coming from others and the need to stay consistent with them all wear you down? Do you fear that you'll fail or that you're just not good enough? Do you compare yourself to others and criticize yourself in any way (looks, weight, accomplishments, income level)? Are you easily frustrated? Would you consider yourself stressed out more than you'd like? Would you call life complex, hard, and overwhelming? Are you living an inauthentic life and missing out on nourishing relationships that can help you manifest your authentic self?

If you said yes to any of these questions, you're not alone. And you're indeed like millions of adults today who walk around wishing they had the secret to a peaceful, healthful existence despite the demands and rigors of modern life. I'm here to share that secret, which has everything to do with gleaning the wisdom of a two-year-old. Put simply, if you can return to the vibrant mentality of a toddler, you can actually build youth back into your cells and function optimally physically, emotionally, spiritually, and in any other way possible. You can also become your truest self. Let me explain.

» A Doctor's Greatest Discovery: What More Than Thirty Years Treating Skin Has Taught Me

At this point you're probably wondering how someone who has made a name for himself in the skincare industry could possibly write a book about overall health and wellness (let alone the fountain of youth). You'd be surprised by what my experience has taught me over the years. The years I spent treating skin were my training grounds for establishing an inclusive approach to health that goes far beyond the surface of the body. And my whole mission—and medical practice—has shifted dramatically since I discovered what I think is today's most pervasive accelerator of aging: cultural stress.

Just what is cultural stress? Cultural stress is proving to be the sneakiest silent killer of all. And it has nothing to do with the everyday stress that acts as background noise in your life or even the acute stress you experience when you're trying to meet a deadline or avoid an accident. Cultural stress is much more insidious. It's what you experience when you're merging onto a congested highway with thoughts of being late again and not having time to check your e-mail before 9 o'clock or respond to the twenty messages marked high-priority from yesterday. (And despite your hyperconnections to others through modern technology, a part of you feels lonely and isolated.) Cultural stress is not the "survival" response that is caused by actual danger. Cultural stress is wearing and tearing us down daily in ways we never thought possible—so much so that I've launched international studies to explore its impact, as well as offered grants to researchers who investigate cultural stress.

Cultural stress enters our lives sooner than we think. As soon as society began to affect you, around the age of three, and you became cognizant—however subconsciously—of your world, you began to age. This phenomenon is the core subject of this book, which may be the most important one I write in my long career. It has taken me nearly forty years to arrive at this simple conclusion that is finally backed by solid science. Most people wrongly assume that I address just skin issues. This couldn't be further from the truth. Today, most of my work entails teaching people how to change their attitudes about themselves first and foremost and build youth from the inside out via a set of practical strategies that can combat cultural stress and simultaneously encourage their cells to behave younger from the inside out—from all the way down in their DNA to the skin that glows on the outside. And this is what I'm going to show you how to do in this book, too.

Although I have devoted my life to making beautiful, healthy skin attainable for everyone and have always rooted my practice in the idea that skincare can lead the way to overall health, skin is a microcosm of the entire body—it reflects what is going on inside. People who come to me experience an evaluation of their health that is unlike any they get in a doctor's office today. Are they happy? Do they have unresolved problems in their lives? Is their stress taking a hidden toll and triggering the physical aging and health challenges that they now have and are prepared to address? Do they feel like they are living truly authentic lives attuned to who they want to be or become?

Case in point: I once had a patient who was very successful in his professional life. He came to me for an evaluation in the hopes I could make him look younger than his fifty-odd years. He seemed to be happy, and he ranked everything an 8 or 9 out of a perfect 10 when I asked him questions about the quality of his life. When I asked him to pick out a mantra among several that I gave him to consider for himself, he chose "Become yourself." This was somewhat surprising to me because I thought he was already "himself" and happy with who he'd become. But then he began talking about the pressures he faced to keep his success going and said that he no longer felt like he was the person he wanted to be. He felt like he lived his life for others and was always at the mercy of other people's needs and expectations rather than his own. At that moment, I knew exactly what was causing all the accelerated aging that was so apparent on his face and that he was so concerned about. When I performed a more in-depth examination of his physical health with the help of standard lab reports, he showed further signs of advanced aging at a cellular level that were well beyond his chronological age.

The manner in which I treat all my patients typically leads to clues I can use to help them acknowledge their own emotional challenges that get in the way of their experience of true health—and looking as youthful as possible. Obviously, I'm not talking about people who have severe clinical depression and who would do well with tradi-tional medicine to treat their illness. I'm referring to the millions of us who walk around dreaming of a better, more fulfilling life where we radiate health from a deeply rooted sense of contentment and peaceful well-being. In fact, when I ask people what the one thing is that will make them happy, they rarely mention money, a better career, or a facelift. Instead, they refer to the holy grail: being 100 percent comfortable and confident with who they are. Isn't that the ultimate goal? I know that for myself, my job today as a doctor who helps people identify with themselves in ways that support health and maximize their potential is what's been my own "becoming." I've become the real me after years of developing my practice, estab-lishing an inclusive health center, and learning from patients and research alike about the true path to wellness.

I treat an enormous array of people, from those who seem to have no reason to complain about feeling and looking older than the calendar says to individuals struggling with persistent conditions that call for constant attention. We all know that chronic illnesses besiege millions today and dominate our health challenges, including insomnia, obesity, chronic pain, arthritis, anxiety disorders, depres-sion, headaches, chronic fatigue, panic anxiety, allergies, irritable bowel and other gastrointestinal problems, and skin disorders such as acne and eczema. Although rarely do patients come to me to treat a chronic condition unrelated to skin, the vast majority of them expe-rience relief from their maladies once they go through my program. It can work in brilliant synch with any other form of treatment with another doctor, including the use of prescriptions. So yes, my prac-tice may be different from that of other doctors, but one thing we increasingly all witness is the growing number of patients suffering from chronic conditions that are often reflected in their skin and that demand to be taken into consideration when we drum up a solution.

» How Skincare Clued Me into the Ultimate Healthcare Secret

About twenty years ago I increasingly realized that I could no longer serve my patients by just playing the role of a traditional dermatologist—diagnosing skin conditions and treating them accordingly. After all, it's pointless to neglect the 80 percent of skin that topical products cannot reach. It's also futile to spot-treat our exterior as if it's not attached to the rest of the body and mind. Treating the skin alone as an isolated component of the body is like using a small brush to touch up the outdoor paint on a house rocked off its foundation and about to crumble under years of neglect and disrepair. So I began to develop another approach, one that could address both the inside and outside to improve the health and appearance of my patients by strengthening *each cell in the body* and helping patients gain control of the cultural stress in their lives. This new way of looking at treatment earned me recognition as the "Father of Internal Skincare." It also opened the door for me to discover the Water Principle, one of the founding principles upon which my philosophy is based and that you'll read about shortly.

In 2007 I opened my new Inclusive Health Center in Los Angeles, a diagnostic and medical spa completely based on an integrative approach that incorporates healing and medical philosophies from all over the world—Western and Eastern practices, nutrition counseling and therapeutic bodywork from leading experts, and comprehensive analysis of every aspect of a person's health: physical, psychological, spiritual, and cultural. I could not have predicted the feedback I got from people about their fantastic life changes just a few months after the opening of my new facility. You'll read about some of them in this book.

Admittedly, this isn't the first time I've written about my discoveries. But it's the first time I've had the advantage of hindsight for long enough to really make bold and declaratory statements about the secrets to aging gracefully and feeling as young as possible each and every year. Since the publication of my last book in 2010, I've noticed a surprising pattern in what predicts those who succeed and those who fail in their attempts to achieve better health. The single most powerful factor in my patients' lives is not the daily skincare regimen they keep nor their attention to diet and exercise; it's their ability to manage cultural stress. When I went back to the scientific data I'd collected over the course of more than ten years of scientific research and from more than four thousand patients following my prescriptions, the results were shouting out to me loud and clear: overcoming cultural stress could be the most essential and effective strategy to sustaining positive changes in well-being, especially with regard to weight loss and overall happiness. The people who shed the most weight, boosted their metabolism and increased their muscle mass the most, improved their looks and skin health, and reported feeling younger and gaining higher self-esteem all had one thing in common: lower levels of cultural stress.[1]

» Controlling Your Genetic Destiny

Over the past couple of years, I even went so far as to put my theory to the test, conducting a pilot genetic study with people who were clearly living under the weight of a lot of cultural stress.[2] Lo and behold, my study found that once they gained control of this stress using the same strategies outlined in this book, they experienced a significant decrease in their cultural stress *at the genetic level*, as measured by changes in the expression of certain genes associated with aging and longevity. That's right: they were able to decrease their body's negative response to cultural stress and enjoy numerous benefits, including turning back the clock on their innate biology and physiology.

So if you're frustrated or unhappy with how you feel and look, whatever your personal health challenges or conditions, then you've come to the right place. Chances are, you picked this book up for a reason. Maybe it's the chronic exhaustion, the lack of a healthy glow, the thinning hair and brittle nails, the extra ten or fifteen pounds you didn't have a year ago, the "older" person looking back at you in the mirror, a recent diagnosis at your doctor's office that scares you, or simply the fear of getting sick and watching your life hit an abysmal ditch. Or perhaps you're among those lucky few who are in excellent health now but you want to do more and learn a fresh approach to preserving your longevity. I'm going to present a revolutionary way to think about taking care of yourself, and you'll soon agree that your frustrations with aging have nothing to do with wrinkles. They go much deeper than that. My hope is that you'll finish this book with a whole different perspective on yourself and your approach to health.

It never ceases to amaze me how my patients have watched their medical problems diminish or in some cases, completely *vanish*. Among the hundreds of thankful letters that I receive routinely from people who've taken my ideas to heart, a singular thought is spoken many different ways: "I feel amazing—better than I've ever felt in my life." Patients share not only how their skin problems have cleared up since they started following my program but how their health—both physical and mental—is changing significantly for the better. *Significantly*. Medical problems are lessening that had not responded to other treatments by other physicians. Excess weight is melting away. Patients report sleeping better, growing stronger hair and nails, and feeling energy they haven't felt in years. Just as I had personally observed changes in my own body while following my own advice, my patients are confirming what I've known for years. Indeed, their bodies are acting younger, and so will yours.

When you begin to take care of yourself, you do a lot more than regain your health and beauty. You build confidence. Self-care helps you take control of your life when it seems off balance. Then you find it transfers to other parts of your life as well. Every person who walks through the doors at my Inclusive Health Center soon realizes this once he or she commences a personalized program. But I know that not everyone can visit my center and participate in all that it has to offer. For this very reason I bring you this book. Just as I do for people at the Inclusive Health Center, I will show you how to take years off your body's age—no matter what your chronological age is. And it will make everyone (including yourself) notice.

CHAPTER 2

The Mystery of Happiness and the Wonder of Water

Water loss is the final common pathway to all aging and disease.

As you can imagine, I'd been living by my principles about health and wellness for decades by the time I reached my seventies. These included practicing the fundamentals of diet and exercise, taking care of my skin, and supporting my emotional self. My principles kept me healthy and happy for the most part, and I knew they worked because I'd taught them to an untold number of people through my work as a professor, lecturer, formulator of products, and clinical doctor. And these individuals were also taking my ideas seriously and reaping the rewards in their well-being. But then something happened: just a few years ago I had an experience that profoundly changed the heart and soul of my principles. It dramatically shifted the way I look at life, interact with others, and approach the entire practice of medicine. And it helped me see everything more clearly and tap a hidden personal potential that I had hardly known existed.

During the fall of 2006 I began to have serious trouble with my eyes. I was on a trip to Hong Kong when I noticed that my vision had suddenly gotten blurry. So I called my wife, Loralee, and asked her to make me an appointment with an eye doctor. The diagnosis was a detached retina, which required corrective surgery. After the operation, I was forced to keep my head down with my chin on my chest for nearly a month while the retina healed. This was painful, and, of course, it forced me to sharply limit my activities. But I had to do it. It was either that or risk losing the vision in the affected eye altogether.

An experience like that would be difficult for anyone, but it was especially hard on me. I've always been a very energetic and active man, so the lack of mobility—not being able to work, exercise, take my long hikes, and follow my usual routine—was, to say the least, challenging. Somehow I had to find an interesting way to fill the hours. It turned out my recuperation became an opportunity to discover a hidden talent. Loralee suggested I use some of the time for art. The previous year, during a stay in Ojai, California, I'd taken an art class for enjoyment. I had never thought of myself as the art type or as someone whose creative instincts leaned in that direction, but we took the class together. It was a very basic lesson and lasted only about an hour. The teacher introduced us to a few materials and techniques and then left us on our own. At the end of the hour I had completed eleven pieces. The teacher glanced at them and said, "I don't recommend you take any formal art classes because they will spoil you. Your style is unique and lessons will ruin it." Clearly, she wanted me to have fun and find time to experiment with art on a regular basis.

Flash-forward about a year. Here I was, cooped up at home with a bad eye and a set of art supplies that I had purchased long ago. They'd never been used. So I fished out the supplies from a closet, sat down at my desk, and started to paint. And paint some more. And some more. The dozens of pieces that I've since created now adorn my office and have been showcased at several institutions, including the University of Southern California. They are constant reminders of this other talent I have that had gone unnoticed for most of my life. They also remind me to stop my typical routine and play with my creativity—just like a kid—once in a while, to color beyond the lines we draw in our adult lives. I sometimes wonder, what else will I discover about myself? Out of a painful and frustrating experience with my eye came this wonderful revelation about myself. And I also started to see the world differently, both literally and metaphorically. It was as if I was now seeing in Technicolor, whereas everything was just black-and-white before.

I've always said the best is yet to come, and I firmly believe in that statement. Not just for me but for everyone who puts a positive effort and attitude forward and reveres one of my most important tenets: be imperfect; live longer. And become free to be yourself. This may be the ultimate path to health and happiness. Put another way, being an emotional youthful person who embraces the power of imperfection and who being that genuine and capable person you really are is the key. It's also the secret to conquering cultural stress.

I'm not equating emotional youthfulness with emotional immaturity. Much to the contrary, I'm referring to the person who is eternally playful, spontaneous, eager to learn something new, unafraid to take risks, unencumbered by fears of failure, and joyful in the company of others. Think about all that you had to learn on your own when you were just figuring out how to crawl, sit up straight, walk, and eventually talk. You went through copious rounds of trial and error. You failed oh-so-many times. And along the way you probably laughed and cried so hard out of sheer bliss or frustration that your belly hurt. When's the last time you had that experience? Those are emotions we all have, but as adults we've learned to hold them in. And as adults, we fall into the perpetual trap of judging ourselves, being overly critical of ourselves, trying to be perfect, and living very controlled lives. We rarely give ourselves permission to say no (like a toddler being defiant!) and instead take on too much in our daily responsibilities.

Is it any wonder we have record rates of depression and chronic illness today? While on the surface there may not seem to be a link between happiness and certain diseases, such as heart disease, obesity, diabetes, and dementia, I think attitude paves our path in all health-related areas. Science is finally revealing just how strong this connection is: over the past decade numerous studies have proven the correlation between a positive outlook and staying healthier as one ages. In one of the most recent longitudinal studies, published in the *Canadian Medical Association Journal* in early 2014, researchers highlighted the detrimental physical effects of negative emotions on the body when they analyzed data on more than three thousand men and women aged sixty and older.[1] About 21 percent were deemed to have a high level of enjoyment of life, 56 percent a medium level, and 23 percent a low level of enjoyment. Over the course of eight years, study participants experienced increasing problems with day-to-day tasks as their mobility declined. About 4 percent of those most upbeat about life developed two or more new functional impairments compared with 17 percent of those who enjoyed life the least. During this time, people who were assessed as enjoying life at a medium or low level were about 80 percent more likely than their happier counterparts to have developed mobility and functional problems.

> Don't focus on the minutia in life. When you come to a wall in the road, life is telling you to make a turn. Go for it.

Even when it comes to stress, which is inevitable and virtually impossible to eradicate, how we deal with and approach that stress is what makes the difference. It's much easier, and more effective, to change your attitude about stress than to change stress's existence. And this has everything to do with our happiness.

» The Mystery of Happiness

What makes people happy? It has been said that an innate feature of the human psyche is to constantly seek self-improvement. Some believe that perhaps one derives happiness within this pursuit. As humans, we are hard-wired to attain happiness and universally yearn to feel it. Because of this, it is logical to conclude that when happiness cannot be achieved, we mourn; we become unhappy. Aristotle believed that happiness is a destination that can be discerned only at the end of life. In his Nichomachean Ethics, he explained that happiness is a measure of virtue, which is realized through the practice of doing ethical, moral works and of amassing "goods" such as health, friendship, and wisdom. Aristotle was also a proponent of achieving a virtuous life through making good decisions and keeping the future in mind. As such, he would not be a fan of today's culture of instant gratification, which he'd view as behavior that's a hindrance to happiness.

Whether you agree or not with Aristotle, the fact remains that happiness is a subjective topic. If it is a destination, then most of us are still trying to find it. However elusive happiness is, countless researchers have attempted to define it, calculate it, describe steps for attaining it, and explain it. Because happiness lacks a universal definition, it's difficult to study. This is perhaps because happiness touches on every aspect of humankind such as our global culture, economics, environment, and relations, as well as other transcendent categories like religion and spirituality. At the individual level, this is also why my multidisciplinary approach to health, which you'll learn about in the next chapter, works.

No doubt happiness is ingrained in the human mind, so much so that whole societies were (and are) built simply to create more for its people. Our forefathers, for instance, wrote in the Declaration of Independence that the pursuit of happiness is a right—one that is bestowed simply because a person has life. And because of this definition, some feel that it requires little self-involvement, that it should just come—and possibly for some, it does. However, for most, work is involved and this work probably includes the removal of barriers that prevent the flow of happiness externally, internally, and emotionally. My approach takes this into account and can be effectively used to remove obstacles that would limit the achievement of happiness and actually encourage the appropriate brain chemistry to promote it.

Happiness can mean something different to different people and cultures around the world. Americans tend to associate happiness with achievements (even though we'd be better off taking pleasure in every minor success, however small or trivial). On the other hand, the Japanese believe happiness is the ability to experience social harmony. The Germans believe happiness is the ability to make good choices. For the people of India, happiness is peace and is defined through family relationships. While some scholars assert that happiness is a measure of income—$75,000 per year, per household in the United States—others have gone so far as to suggest that happiness can be measured through a country's gross domestic product (GDP), though sometimes wealthy nations rank the least happiest as we'll see shortly.[2] Clearly, higher income does not necessarily mean higher well-being, especially once the $75,000 threshold is surpassed.

Happiness does not require luxury. Happiness means finding beauty every day.

In contrast to the belief that GDP is an indicator of happiness, French president Nicolas Sarkozy, in 2009, proposed that his country and others replace the GDP figure with the idea of a gross domestic happiness (GDH) measure—a socioeconomic development metric that accounts for factors such as healthcare availability, leisure time, subjective happiness, and sustainability. Following France's lead, Britain began compiling, in May 2011, a national happiness index, a move that many psychotherapists have lauded as mentally more healthy. Interestingly, the original idea of GDH came from Bhutan in 1972 from then king Jigme Singye Wangchuck, who based his concept on Buddhist principles. It's difficult to be specific on what exactly the GDH metric examines. It has been said to analyze seven areas of wellness including categories such as economic, environmental, physical, mental, workplace, social, and political wellness, but there remains no exact measure.

In another attempt to find the happiest places on earth, the Gallup Organization ranked a list of 148 countries and areas that were examined in 2011. The results are based on five questions that have to do with whether one experienced a lot of enjoyment the day before the survey and whether he or she felt respected, well-rested, laughed and smiled a lot, and did or learned something interesting. The following list shows where the most positive people reside in the world. We didn't make the top twenty (we're number thirty-three, and there were several ties). Note, too that residents of Panama, which ranks 90th in the world with respect to GDP per capita, are among the most likely to report positive emotions. People who live in Singapore, however, are the least likely to report positive emotions— and Singapore ranks fifth in the world in terms of GDP per capita.[3]

1. Panama
1. Paraguay
3. El Salvador
3. Venezuela
5. Trinidad and Tobago
5. Thailand
7. Guatemala
7. Philippines
9. Ecuador
9. Costa Rica
11. Canada

11. Columbia
11. Malaysia
11. Netherlands
11. Ireland
16. Denmark
16. Kuwait
16. Oman
16. Indonesia
16. Honduras

I'm not surprised that most Americans don't claim to be the happiness people on the planet. I witness the unhappiness daily in my work with patients. It's achingly palpable. And it stems from all kinds of issues—work stress, family strife, illness, divorce, death of a loved one, loneliness, and, of course, cultural stress, a real phenomenon we'll explore in chapter 3.

I should point out, however, that other methods of evaluating happiness across various cultures and countries have arrived at better results for us Americans. In 2014, the Organization for Economic Co-operation and Development (OECD) released its latest "Better Life Index," which ranks countries according to eleven criteria it considers essential for a happy life. These include data on health, education, income, and environment. The survey also takes into consideration people's responses about their priorities in life and evaluates their "sense of happiness." Here are the top ten countries:[4]

1. Australia
2. Norway
3. Sweden
4. Denmark
5. Canada
6. Switzerland
7. U.S.
8. Finland

9. Netherlands
10. New Zealand

We as humans are by nature compassionate beings capable of manipulating the way we interact with our environment and how we perceive our experiences. As such, we work hard, attempt to deflect conflict, seek to maintain stability, and perhaps spend most of our time chasing desires, whether external, internal, or emotional. There is something to be said for those who "learn" to be happy or who work through processes to cognitively create their happiness. But whether happiness is a biologically controlled function, a learned state of mind, or a cognitive process remains the subject of countless studies, with pharmaceutical companies leading the way on the biological studies.

The Happiness Test

Which of the following makes people happier?
- Making more money.
- Finding a soul mate.
- Losing ten pounds.
- Moving into a new house.
- Achieving success.
- Having better genes; happiness is genetic, just like the color of one's eyes and hair.

Answer: None of the above is true. New science proves that happiness is a process—not a goal. And it's not necessarily about having fun either. As I clearly stated in *The Water Secret* based on research, happiness is about 50 percent genetic, 40 percent intentional, and 10 percent circumstantial.[5] That 40 percent category—the intentional one—is the most important. Circumstances can change, or you can become accustomed to them (e.g., a new car, a bigger house, a promotion) such that they no longer make you happy. On the other hand, when you are engaged in a life purpose that has meaning to you, which can be anything from rearing children to doctoring the elderly in underserved areas, happiness finds you in the way you live and look at the world. In other words, happiness is more a choice than an outcome or destination. It's an action, not a result.

The reality is that happiness is probably a combination of all three elements—biological, learned, and cognitive—and this is what my approach to wellness honors. How much is biological, learned, or cognitive is unknown, but when people use my three-step program, this is irrelevant. And I think we can all agree that regardless of how each one of us defines happiness, it's a state of mind and its destination is the brain.

» Turning Back the Clock through the Water Principle

While studying happiness from a purely scientific perspective may be hard, it's not as challenging to study aging. And everyone has an opinion in this realm. Years ago, I myself started looking for the most comprehensive approach to understanding health, aging, and happiness. Theories about chronic inflammation and free-radical damage, among countless others, weren't enough for me. (The last time I checked, I found more than three hundred ideas on the causes of aging.) In 2009, the Nobel Prize in Physiology or Medicine was awarded to three Americans whose experiments were pivotal in our understanding of telomeres, the protective coverings on the ends of chromosomes that impact cell division. The amount of the substance in the body that builds telomeres, called telomerase, ultimately influences cell death and, in the larger scheme of life, aging.

But none of these theories paint the whole picture for me, as they are like plot twists in the mystery book of life. Certainly these biological events and substances play a proven role, but I sense that they do so within a much larger and universal context.

So with every idea that emerged on aging, at the back of my mind continued to sound the famous words from the Nobel Laureate in Medicine Albert Szent-Györgyi von Nagyrapolt: "Discovery is seeing what everybody has seen and thinking what nobody else has thought." And even though I've led plenty of pioneering studies about the importance of controlling inflammatory pathways and nourishing the body with good ingredients, I've always felt something was missing. I equate the situation to a house with a caved-in roof after a light rain: it does no good to replace the roof if you don't take care of what really brought it down in the first place, such as termites that weakened the structure before the storm hit. In the body, if you're not addressing root causes of disorders and disease, or the triggers of inflammation, you're not going to support the body's inherent healing powers to maintain a strong and robust body.

By the time I started painting and embracing the gifts of imperfection, I had already built my health center. Adding the importance of emotional youthfulness was the finishing touch on my whole philosophy. It further allowed me to understand the aging process and teach what I believe has become my most important contribution to science: the Water Principle. Let me briefly take you back to the events that led up to my theory, for my discovery didn't happen in a lab or other traditional medical setting. As with many scientific breakthroughs, it evolved slowly over time as I tried to understand my patients and gather evidence from them. It's amazing what you can learn from patients when you delve into their habits and personal "secrets" to staying young, especially when you witness tens of thousands pass through your office from all walks of life. Some seem to defy their age as if by magic while others show clear signs of having jumped too far ahead into the future before their time. Genetics and luck aside ("luck" meaning avoiding diseases like cancer or other serious illnesses of unknown origin), I saw clear patterns among those who were aging exceptionally well and those who looked desperate for a reboot.

One patient in particular has always stood out in my mind. When Ted walked into my office more than a decade ago, he was in supreme health for a man of his eighty-eight years. He never got sick. He hiked every day, stayed active in community events and organizations, had a positive outlook on life even though he'd lost his wife a few years previously, and enjoyed a healthy diet that included eggs every other day. Ted may have had a good set of genes, but I knew that his chosen lifestyle dictated how well he lived more than anything else. He was just one of thousands who offered me insights into aging well, and I took his wisdom to heart. After all, I myself was looking for the recipe to feeling and looking as vibrant as possible. Patients like Ted helped me see where I could make improvements and then share that knowledge with others.

One feature that emerged from my gleanings was the fact that my healthiest patients shared the ability to hold water without the classic "water retention" in the wrong areas. In other words, they were well hydrated (and looked it) yet were not bloated and did not have to lug around bottles of water all day. My own experience as an avid hiker who continually felt dehydrated on strenuous climbs inspired me to think in a new way about how to encourage my cells to hold more water. I theorized that the water conserving strength of the cell's membrane—its ability to keep water *inside the cell* (hence, *cellular* water)—was the fundamental marker of health and youthful vitality. The diets of my healthiest patients like Ted were rife with the very nutrients that make up cellular membranes, the outer yet permeable boundary of a cell that envelops its interior and allows certain molecules to enter or exit the cell.

> *Life can be described as a process during which the highly hydrated state of fertilized oocytes, embryos, newborns, toddlers, and so on, is transformed into a gradually more and more dehydrated one.*

Eager to translate this theory into practice, I used my background as a pharmacist and a physician to attack the problem of cellular water loss. I naturally became the first case study as I experimented on myself by taking various nutrients in the hopes of creating an ideal environment for maintaining the building blocks of healthy cells. This included supplementing my diet with antioxidant minerals, vitamins, and plant-based compounds; adding anti-inflammatory agents to the mix to prevent free radicals from forming in the first place; and finally throwing in some omega fats to draw more water to the cells. (And, like Ted, I started to eat eggs every other day.) My weekly hikes afforded me the perfect testing grounds.

Flash-forward several years. By the mid-1990s, I was convinced enough of my theory from my own experience to share it with a few hundred patients whose health needed a boost. Not to my surprise, I found that those who took advantage of my internal care program felt better, slept better, and had a remarkable reduction in the severity of common skin disorders such as dryness, acne, and cellulite. I also found that their skin had an apparent increase in structural strength and resilience that made it appear firmer, plumper, brighter—more like young skin. And I knew, as every dermatologist knows, that the outer appearance reflected what was going on inside.

With the help of new technologies that were emerging to measure cellular integrity and patients' bodily ratio of water *outside* their cells versus *inside* their cells, I further validated my theory. The people who had robust cellular water content were overall healthier. And I noted clear parallels between aspects of the individuals' lives that contributed to health or, conversely, ill health, and their cellular water. Someone who was sick or unhappy didn't show a lot of cellular water. On the other hand, people with outward signs of health and well-being and who maintained healthy lifestyle habits scored high in the cellular water department. They were also the happiest, despite difficult life circumstances.

By the year 2000, I'd hired a research staff and put my theory through more rigorous testing both in the lab and in a clinical setting. I also put patients through my three-part program to see if I could change their cellular water for the better and improve their health.

Lo and behold, thousands of people did indeed transform their lives in uniquely individual ways just by following my simple protocol. Take Monica, a thirty-eight-year-old type 2 diabetic who came to me with a persistent case of acne. After a month following my program alongside a specific treatment for her acne, her blood sugar stabilized and her acne cleared. Or consider Stewart, a fifty-seven-year-old man suffering with depression largely due to the ongoing pain of rheumatoid arthritis. He adopted my strategies and three months later found that his arthritis pain was considerably reduced and his depression was lifting. And I'll never forget Jessica, a twenty-nine-year-old woman already burned out from her job as vice president of publicity for a large corporation. She looked ten years older and was already complaining of advanced aging. Ten weeks later, after following my program, she felt like she had reclaimed her life. (And she looked *younger* than twenty-nine, believe it or not.)

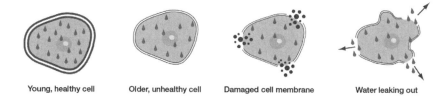

Young, healthy cell   Older, unhealthy cell   Damaged cell membrane   Water leaking out

The Water Principle

So I knew that my program was working, but then in 2012 I upped the ante on my investigations further by conducting a genetic study.[6] This really put my program to the test. Although it was a very small study, involving six women, the results spoke volumes. It compared blood and skin biopsies collected at the start of the program and after twelve weeks and again at twenty-four weeks. We examined changes in certain genes known to be big players in aging, such as those responsible for DNA repair, the birth of new cells, metabolism, fat burning, and immunity. And what we found surprised even me:

the simple lifestyle modifications I had these women make led to significant changes at the molecular level, which resulted in their bodies acting and behaving much younger than their chronological age. We were also able to confirm what I'd long thought to be true: health could be measured by how strongly the cells were holding water. The results indicated that the women's genes were expressing themselves in positive ways thanks to well-hydrated cells. In other words, they were less susceptible to disease.

Moreover, these women, who ranged in age from forty-six to fifty-three, were uniquely vulnerable to depression at the start of the program. In fact, on average they had a 33 percent lifetime risk of suffering from depression based on certain laboratory measurements. (In the general population, one's average risk is about 16 percent.) But after just twelve weeks, they had reduced their levels of risk by nearly 20 percent.

While you might think these lifestyle modifications were all about diet and exercise (e.g., chewing on raw kale and using a treadmill), that's far from the case. At the core of the program was what I've been talking about since the beginning of the book: tapping the power of imperfection and gaining control of the cultural stress in their lives. This, it turns out, has a huge say in your body's ability to turn back its clock and turn on its youth genes. These women harnessed the power of maximizing the 40 percent of happiness that's under one's control and reaped big rewards that could be clinically measured. And contrary to what you might think, they didn't do it just by switching up their diets and taking daily walks. By the time I was treating this group of women and taking them through my program, I knew that among the most powerful things I could do for them at the start was share my words of inspiration. Over recent years, I've amassed a library of insights that I use with patients, finding that they help encourage people to make the initial shift in attitude that can then open the door to a new, better life. The results I was getting from these insights alone were helping me make the ultimate connection between my theory of aging and the impact of emotional health on maintaining robust, hydrated cells. In addition to sprinkling my insights throughout the book, I have listed them in appendix A and invite you to read through them to find ones that resonate with you. Read them aloud to yourself and really think about them. In general, these insights encourage you to think the way you thought as a toddler and to become your authentic self.

Your Wellspring

Despite what your high school biology text taught you, you are *not* 75 to 80 percent water. You once were—long ago when you were a babbling baby fresh from your mother's watery womb. But now you're closer to 50 percent water. What happened? Well, you've aged, and since your early years, internal and external factors have damaged your cells and weakened their ability to retain water. This explains the signs of aging that probably emerged in your late twenties or (if you were lucky) early thirties: your skin began to become drier, fine lines and wrinkles appeared, your sleep patterns changed, your flexibility took a hit, your digestion slowed, and your energy wavered. You started to complain about more aches and pains, need more caffeine to get through your day, and have a tougher time keeping excess weight off. No, this didn't happen overnight, although it may have seemed that way one random day when you "suddenly" noted all these changes in a mirror, on a scale, or in your doctor's office.

What's been going on has been a slow, inevitable decline in your cells' capacity to hold water for good use. If you drank a gallon of water a day and I called you dehydrated, would you believe me? Probably not. But it's true: unless your cells can retain the water they require to support cellular functions, then drinking all the water in the world won't make much of a difference (and you'll need to keep drinking). Every part of the body, from your brain to the tendons and ligaments in your feet, needs water to function properly. Without enough water in their cells, organs cannot perform their normal operations or communicate with each other.

Which brings me to another fact that goes against the grain of conventional wisdom: not all water is created equal. As you've probably figured out by now, your body contains two types of water: *wellness water* inside your cells and *wastewater* floating in between your cells, the kind that will age you and make you feel fat and sluggish. Puffy eyes, swollen ankles, and a bloated stomach, for example, are all examples of extracellular waste fluid and signs that the body isn't handling water efficiently. Cell damage can occur anywhere, including in the blood vessels, heart, skin, liver, and muscles. Picture a blood vessel that's as strong and sturdy as a brand-new hose. Now picture that same hose riddled with microscopic holes, leaking water. That water escapes and becomes waste.

Wellness water, on the other hand, sustains cellular activities and thus life; this is what allows you to remain healthy, trim, and beautiful. The caveat, of course, is to keep water where it's supposed to be if cells are somehow compromised and porous as an outcome of aging. First, you have to sew up the cracks, and then you have to ensure you're getting high-quality water, which you won't necessarily find in a bottle or faucet. You'll shortly come to understand what I mean, as I take you through my "Pitcher of Health" and train you to choose foods and beverages that optimize your hydration.

When patients ask me to explain how such a focus on water could be so critical, I offer another perspective: you've gone from being a glass nearly full with water when you were born to a glass that's half empty. And a glass that's half empty can't handle the rigors of daily life as well, from those pesky free radicals that swarm in response to certain lifestyle habits and exposure to UV rays and pollution to chronic inflammation or any other factor that accelerates the aging process. I often find myself fielding questions about inflammation, a concept that has been running rampant in scientific circles lately. Billions of dollars and the most brilliant minds in the world have been unraveling the mystery of how inflammation causes your body to self-destruct. But this has caused much confusion among the public, who now seem to think it's a disease itself.

Inflammation is routinely advertised as something bad for you. The truth is, inflammation is a warning sign that the body is trying to heal itself. It's key to survival. And it's far from a disease. Inflammation, in fact, is a *symptom*—a sign of something else going on in the body that ushers in the inflammatory response for help. Think of it as our body warring against harmful agents, an indication that the body is in the process of repairing itself. You would die without an inflammatory response. It's critical to the immune system. It tells us our immune system is working. If we never had inflammation, no action would occur in the dynamic cellular immune system network to offer assistance within the body. When we know this, it becomes clear that inflammation in a healthy body, when it's not an overreaction, chronic, or irreparable, really results in increased general health because of the repair process that's happening at the cellular level.

Here's a prime example to explain: when you cut your finger, the inflammation process begins, ultimately to spur the healing. Once the skin is healed, the inflammation goes away. In the case of more serious forms of inflammation, such as heart disease, the same holds true. If you were to take care of the underlying cause of the heart disease—chronic high blood pressure and plaque formation on the arterial walls, for example—then the inflammation would go away and so would the disease. It's very difficult, if not impossible, to "treat" inflammation. You have to treat the *causes* of inflammation. But treating all the causes of aging is a mighty tall order. What if you could address what happens as a result of the aging process and then essentially reverse-engineer the treatment? That's what the Water

Principle does. Because the Water Principle offers a unifying theory that helps us make sense of the aging process, it tells us *how to slow it down*—and in some cases *reverse* it—from a singular focal point. What's more, it reveres the body as a whole. We all have multiple issues to deal with when it comes to health, which is why an inclusive approach is ideal.

Regardless of what causes aging or disease, the final common pathway is the reduction of water in our tissues. Yes, we can say life is simply a slow process of continual dehydration. We wilt and wither over time, just like that plant you forgot to water until it was too late. Even Hippocrates, the father of medicine, thought of the human body in terms of four main climate-like categories more than twenty-three centuries ago: humid, dry, warm, and cold. He said when we are young, we are humid and warm, and when we age, these two factors no longer prevail—the body moves into the dry and cold categories, which eventually dominate. As our cells lose their integrity, we become more vulnerable to all the aspects of aging, such as oxidative stress (free radicals), inflammation, psychological and cultural stress, and disease. It's a vicious cycle: our cells and connective tissues hold less and less water as we age, and we age as a result of that inability to hold on to water.

One of the easiest ways to remember the power of the Water Principle is to think of driving a car across the country. You'll encounter some tough terrain along the way, including dirt roads, bumps, and steep inclines. If your tires get little holes in them, they will hold less air and the engine will have to work harder to go the distance. The car will become fuel inefficient as it chugs along, demanding more work from other parts of the car to keep going. Eventually that extra-hard work begins to exhaust your transmission and the car begins to slowly fall apart. A good set of tires can make all the difference. And so can a good set of body cells. Everything about you will benefit.

Weight Loss, Not Water Retention

One question I often get soon after explaining the Water Principle is whether or not people who follow it gain weight due to water retention. True?

Not so fast. In fact, the opposite is true: people who live by the Water Principle *lose* weight as their bodies become more efficient. You will weigh more if the water is in the wrong place—like puffy eyes or swollen ankles. Water in your cells not only allows you to function at a higher level but also increases your basal metabolism rate so you burn even more calories at rest to lose more unhealthy weight. Here's another way to look at it: as your cells become more hydrated, they function optimally and utilize more energy. In all my studies of people following the Water Principle, the one common thread among patients is a heightened metabolism and a reduction in body fat.

Integrative, Preventive, or Inclusive Health

It's amazing to me how many resources we have at our fingertips these days and yet we continue to battle chronic diseases. We have the wonder of powerful new drugs on the market, access to the best medicine that money can buy, spa-like retreats sprinkled throughout the country, and the knowledge to tell the difference between what's good and not so good for us. Yet we aren't all functioning at our best and feeling and looking the best we can be. We're still not 100 percent healthy. Why is this happening?

"Integrative medicine" and "preventive medicine" have become buzzwords in the last decade. We seem to think that these practices help solve our health problems, but they, in fact, perpetuate another problem: focusing on a single condition or disease. Take, for example, heart disease, which is the leading killer in America. If you are a heart patient, chances are you'll be taking medications prescribed by a traditional doctor. You'll be told to watch your diet and avoid unhealthy fats that can clog your arteries. You may even be recommended to an acupuncturist known for heart-healthy treatments.

That's all fine and good, but it still puts the focus on a single organ, your heart. What about your stress level and emotional health that's contributing to high blood pressure? What if you've got an undiagnosed problem festering in your lungs or brain that's exacerbating your heart condition? This is akin to not seeing the forest for the trees.

What I love about the Water Principle is that it not only regards the health of the whole individual but does so by considering every single cell in the body. When every cell functions at its highest level, the body's environment is optimized for the health of every organ and system—not just one. So let's take, for example, the theory about telomeres again for a moment. Like plastic tips on the ends of shoelaces, telomeres sheathe the ends of chromosomes to keep them from "fraying" and losing their genetic content. Without telomeres, the chromosomes and the genes they hold would come apart. Telomeres are necessary for cells to divide and are involved in directing the number of divisions. In essence, telomeres have a say in cell life (or death) and how well we age. So how can you protect your telomeres?

Well, think about it. Telomeres are part of a cell. To protect our telomeres, we have to protect our cells. We have to preserve normal cellular functioning. And that is exactly the goal of the Water Principle. Another way to think about it is to see the Water Principle as the means by which we gain control of our cellular health. It supports optimal functioning of *all* cellular roles, from maintaining telomeres and encouraging cell division to reducing dangerous inflammation and removing waste products and pathogens. It acknowledges and values both the forest *and* the trees, so to speak.

Hence, "inclusive health" relates to the whole body and all its trillions of cells. Wouldn't you rather address every single cell in your body than treat just a cluster in your heart or liver or brain? Everything in your body is connected. Though it's become customary to see your heart, for example, as operating separately from your brain, both are inextricably linked. So are your toes and eyes, and your kidneys and ears. It's time for a new—inclusive—perspective. If you can begin to view your health in an inclusive manner, then you've already taken a huge leap. Now you just have to follow through and learn how to take care of yourself inclusively.

Most people falsely accept signs of aging such as weight gain, fatigue, and familial patterns of disease as inevitable. The truth: Upwards of 80 percent of longevity is attributed to *lifestyle*—not your encoded DNA. I see this fact played out every day in my practice and have done so for the past thirty years. Even when it comes to the risk of getting cancer, lifestyle plays a much bigger role. The vast majority of women (70 to 80 percent) who are diagnosed with breast cancer, for example, do not have a family history of the disease.

As soon as we're born, aging begins. With every birthday, new symptoms emerge—a new face line here, a stiffer joint there. And when we aren't careful, this inevitable decline accelerates. The door to illness and disease widens. None of us can escape aging. It's a certainty that Benjamin Franklin neglected to add to his short list alongside death and taxes. The anti-aging market has fueled the skincare and spa industries for decades as aging individuals continue to seek new roads to youth. And it's not just youth in looks but more importantly youth in how they feel. No one likes to feel lousy even if all looks relatively good on the outside.

> By the time you reach fifty, your lifestyle determines 80 percent of your aging process. The difference between a sixty-year-old who looks forty-something and a forty-year-old who looks sixty is maintenance. But it's never too late to turn back the clock physically and from a cellular standpoint.

If you don't have your health, nothing else—not even a youthful appearance—really matters.

In the 1980s, when I introduced alpha hydroxy acids to the

professional skincare industry, women flocked to their estheticians to exfoliate away their top wrinkly layers. As years passed, we found better vehicles for our ingredients. At my company, we discovered the power of stable vitamin C used in an anhydrous silicone formula and other topical antioxidants, and we started to see remarkable improvements in skin. But there were limitations on how much skin could improve. Regardless of what we did on the outside to maintain the results, and no matter how much sun protection was used, we continued to see the gradual changes from aging creep in. It was clear that skin aging involves more than just external influences, so research would have to go beyond skin's outermost layers. These were still the days when estheticians, doctors, and lifestyle practitioners followed their own divergent paths without considering the value of sharing knowledge or collaborating.

As I noted earlier, my own search for new approaches to help my patients led me to create an interdisciplinary approach to skincare. I had to look beneath the surface of the skin and examine the relationship of the internal aspects of the body—unfolding the mechanisms of inflammation, disease, and hormones—to the health of the skin. My research confirmed what I knew instinctively: making changes in internal health and emotional composition, in addition to therapeutic skin treatments, produced profound results in not just skin health, but total health. Moreover, my continuing work with the Water Principle showed me, through direct clinical examination, that the key to longevity, youth, and health is found at the cellular level.

In my quest to find the next "it" ingredient or method that would take us to new levels of rejuvenation, I was faced with the grim reality that there really is no way to stop aging. In fact, if you were to ask different scientists what it means to "age," you'll get different answers. We don't even have a clear definition of what that verb means. The only thing that stops aging assuredly is death. Aging has perplexed humans for millennia, and scientists have explored cellular aging ad nauseam. In the process, researchers have presented more than three hundred theories on the causes of aging. It's difficult to say which theory is correct and which is not, as the answer may stem from a combination of theories—and new theories will no doubt continue to emerge. Free radicals and inflammation, for example, tell only part of the story.

All these theories on aging aside, on closer inspection, a distinct and undeniable pattern emerges. It seems the largest clue to solving the mystery of aging starts small, at the cellular level, and simply with life's most natural and valuable element, water, as the key. When our cells are not fully hydrated, they cannot function at optimal levels, and this leads to aging. When cells deteriorate, disorders, diseases, and death occur. Studies show that the elderly, especially if diseased, have low levels of water inside their cells. My own studies of people at both ends of the spectrum—those in poor health and those in supreme health—also show distinct differences in their cellular water content. Hence, the net effect of aging is cellular water loss—which, as you know by now, is the foundation of the Water Principle.

» The Science of Aging

Think of your body as composed of two components: cells and connective tissue. Both harbor and use water to sustain life, so in a sense you can think of your body as made up of cells, connective tissue, and water. That's it.

Cells make up your muscles and organs, including your skin. Though skin cells are not the same as, say, heart cells, their basic traits are the same. All cells have a protective membrane composed of fats (lipids) and lecithin, a natural antioxidant and emollient found in all living organisms that's essential to cell membranes. Within the cell membrane is a substance called cytoplasm, and within the cytoplasm is the cell's nucleus. The nucleus is the control center of the cell, and damage to a cell's outer membrane is as lethal to the cell as direct damage to its nucleus. Both the cytoplasm and the nucleus are predominantly made up of water. Your heart, brain, bones, and outer skin layer are all made up of cells.

Connective tissue is the fibrous material that binds your muscles and organs in place and connects one organ to another. This tissue has very few cells and contains what's called the body's matrix, which is a semisolid matter made of materials such as hyaluronic acid, a water-loving substance that can actually attract up to one thousand times its weight in water. Collagen and elastin, two structural proteins you'll learn more about later in this chapter, keep the connective tissue firm and hold its shape. You get the tools you need to manufacture collagen and elastin from the amino acids in the foods you eat. Blood vessels, nerves, tendons, ligaments, and your internal layers of skin are all connective tissue.

As we age, our cells and connective tissue break down. They lose the ability to attract and hold on to all the water they need to function at their best, like they do in a baby's new body. The water that seeps out wanders aimlessly through the spaces between cells and connective tissue. This, as you know by now, is what I call wastewater.

Not only is wastewater useless, but it can cause problems. It can build up in inconvenient ways, leaving you with puffy ankles or eyelids. Your body can be full of this wastewater and still be dehydrated because the water can't reach the cells and connective tissues where it's

What happens when you age?

- Wrinkles
- Sun damage
- Less hair in some places, more in others
- Poor memory
- Lack of sleep
- Lack of energy
- Poor digestion
- Reduced circulation
- More stress
- Chronic disease
- And more

needed most and where it keeps your heart, lung, brain, liver, and skin healthy and vital. Can anything be done about this wastewater?

Absolutely. First, it helps to understand what factors in to this water loss and then take steps to reduce that buildup of wastewater by repairing your cell membranes and strengthening the structure of the connective tissue.

Only one word describes what happens over time—"aging"—but this process actually has different reasons and triggers. Let's take a look at the three main types of aging. This will help you to completely grasp how to take control of the process.

Intrinsic Aging: A Fact of Life

Indeed, part of aging is just that—aging. It's simply a natural process that happens no matter what you do to halt it. It's what would occur had you never been in the sun, swallowed toxins, taken a stressful exam, smoked a cigarette, partied past your bedtime, breathed metropolitan air, and so on. It's what would occur despite living in a bubble and getting Botox till your face is stone cold. Genetics play a key role in intrinsic aging. If your parents aged well, odds are, you will too. In the body, intrinsic aging results in a loss of collagen and elastin and a reduction of water in the cells.

Don't deal with what you could have done. Deal with what you are going to do.

Environmental Aging: Inevitable but Controllable

Extrinsic aging is also known as "environmental aging," a term I introduced back in 1993. Extrinsic or environmental aging is exactly what it sounds like: aging from the combination of injury to your outsides and compromised cellular functions on your insides. Luckily, this is the type of aging that we can control to some degree. Factors such as excessive sun exposure, pollution, smoking, stress, poor diet, and intake of drugs or alcohol contribute to this type of aging.

The classic signs of environmental aging are usually written all over a person's skin in the form of redness, dryness, thinner skin, sagging and wrinkles, and hyperpigmentation (e.g., "age spots"). You probably can't see the water loss in the cells, but it's there. The good news is, the effects of environmental aging can be minimized through both preventive actions and treatment.

Hormonal Aging: Another Fact of Life

Hormonal aging has gained tremendous attention in recent years and has no doubt spurred much conversation, especially in women's circles. Hormonal aging occurs as levels of estrogen decline, which starts happening long before menopause. In fact, by the time a woman reaches her twenties, she will have begun to age and her skin will probably show it. The reasons why this happens vary and include many factors such as stress and lifestyle.

Hormonal aging in men, called andropause, can also occur as levels of testosterone decline. It is less talked about in general but the effects in men are also widely visible when you consider the hallmark signs: sagging breasts (which is pronounced if they are overweight), excessive hair growth in atypical spots such as the ears and eyebrows, and thinning hair on top of the head.

Just as testosterone is present in both men and women, so is estrogen. In men, estrogen is made in small amounts as a by-product of the testosterone conversion process. This estrogen helps support bones, a healthy libido and heart, and brain function. As with women, age can precipitate an imbalance of men's natural hormones. Too much estrogen, for example, can reduce the levels of testosterone and trigger a loss of muscle tone and sexual function. It can also cause fatigue and increased body fat.

Although the eventual dryness and inelasticity of skin that come with age are inevitable facts of life, the aging process is a cumulative one that occurs at varying rates from individual to individual. Hormonal aging does not turn on like a light switch; rather, it's like a dimmer that slowly brightens as one's chronological age progresses, and the speed at which it brightens is different from person to person. Most women are all too familiar with the ravages of low estrogen levels: weakening of the collagen and elastin fibers makes them look old as their skin becomes thinner and more fragile. Adding insult to injury, facial hair and breakouts increase, and water content in their cells decreases. In short, they don't look like a glowy youth anymore, and nothing is more frustrating than the combination of dry skin *and* acne.

So why does this loss of estrogen lead to so many skin-damaging effects? Estrogen is your skin's best friend. It helps prevent aging in three big ways: it prevents a decrease in skin collagen in postmenopausal women; it increases the skin's collagen content, which maintains skin thickness; and it helps skin maintain moisture by promoting the production of certain substances in the skin that boost hydration.

Because everything in the body is connected, shifts in hormones through the years can have profound effects on the body. Hormones are simply chemical messengers that travel in the body's blood vessels to target areas where they have an intended effect. The chemical messages, which are tiny in volume, have many large and important jobs such as regulating metabolism, mood, growth and development, and tissue function. The body's hormonal system includes the sex glands (testes in men, ovaries in women), the kidneys, the pancreas, the hypothalamus and the pituitary, pineal, parathyroid, thyroid, and adrenal glands. In addition to estrogen, the most familiar hormones include progesterone, cortisol, adrenaline, and androgens like testosterone. Every organ has certain hormones, and many hormones have multiple functions that overlap. When all hormones are balanced, the body works as it should, organs function properly, tissues are supple and resilient, and skin is youthful. Conversely, the smallest variation in hormone levels can cause great, catastrophic effects all over the body and on the skin.

While the study of menopause-related skin issues began in the mid-1990s, well before then I noted many hormonal skin patterns that exist in women. As I began to isolate certain factors and sift through my data, I was startled to find some direct correlations between hormones and skin conditions. While the term "menopausal skin" became quite popular as some of my contemporaries believed that menopause marked the beginning of skin issues due to hormone decline and imbalance, I knew this to be false based on my patients and hands-on experience.

The truth is, as we age, so do our organs and glands. In women, estrogen and progesterone production declines. And as I just stated, hormonal aging does not just happen once a woman reaches menopause. The true beginning of hormonal aging occurs decades before menopause sets in and continues to occur well after menopause.

Unlike environmental aging, for which we know clear and wise lifestyle strategies to prevent and reduce it, hormonal aging is most troublesome to treat effectively. It requires an inclusive approach and a great understanding of the body's systems and complex interactions. That said, I won't ask you to learn all those systems and symphonic interactions. By following the three-step program outlined in part 2, you'll be putting into practice the very methods to heal and control hormonal aging. This is incredibly important because one of the chief side effects of hormonal aging is a decline in cellular immunity. As dried-out, aging cells lose their ability to renew themselves and operate properly, their functionality slows down—similar to a used piece of equipment that doesn't work like new. For this reason, women approaching menopause or beyond it become more susceptible to cardiovascular disease, cancer, hypothyroidism, polycystic ovarian syndrome, autoimmune disorders, high blood pressure, obesity, insulin resistance, and more. They become vulnerable to a bevy of health challenges.

Die Late, Not Old

All humans experience a combination of the three types of aging to certain degrees. Despite the fact that hormonal aging is the most troublesome to address effectively, fundamentally it and the other two types of aging can be addressed with one simple element—water.

What I love about the Water Principle is that it offers a unifying theory that helps us make sense of the aging process. It tells us how to slow that process down—and in some cases reverse it—from a singular focal point. If water is addressed at the cellular level, then all skin and body issues can be managed more completely.

Why is this so revolutionary? Because for the past century we've been focused on disease treatment and studying diseases on a case-by-case basis. Only recently has science turned to slowing the biological processes of aging as a way to prevent and fight a multitude of diseases. Some still think of cancer, atherosclerosis, osteoporosis, osteoarthritis, immune dysfunction, and skin aging as unrelated. But that insular way of thinking is beginning to change. Until recently, in fact, the notion of reversing human aging was a mere fantasy, absent any scientific support. In the last few years, scientists have gained tremendous grounds on demystifying the aging process and how to manipulate it—forward or backward.

In 2008, for instance, a group of aging experts from both the United States and United Kingdom reported in the prestigious *British Medical Journal* that slowing aging is the best way to combat diseases in the twenty-first century.[7] In other words, the traditional medical approach of attacking individual diseases—cancer, diabetes, heart disease, Alzheimer's disease, Parkinson's disease, and so on— will soon become less effective if we don't determine how all these diseases either interact or share common mechanisms with aging. It's true that middle-aged and older people are most often impacted by simultaneous but independent health problems, a condition technically known as comorbidity. I'll see a sixty-five-year-old man with diabetes, high blood pressure and cholesterol, arthritis, gastric reflux, and a history of depression. The number of medications he's taking is mind-boggling. Or picture an elderly woman suffering from at least ten different ailments and juggling an expensive, confusing cocktail of medications every day. What's more, she's been prescribed other medications, but they cause intolerable side effects, and the more drugs she takes, the greater the risk of dangerous drug interactions. Her predicament is not an unusual one.

Two-thirds of people over age sixty-five and almost three-quarters of people over eighty have multiple chronic health conditions, and the majority of Medicare spending goes to people who have five or more chronic diseases.[8] As a group, these patients fare poorly by any measure. They stay in hospitals longer, experience more serious health complications that could have been prevented, and die younger than patients with less complex medical profiles. Sadly, they are often not treated as whole human beings. Medicine attempts to spot-treat each complicated medical problem to no avail because medicine cannot yet see the forest for the trees.

The authors of the study published in the *British Medical Journal* point out that a cure for any of the major fatal diseases would have only a marginal impact on life expectancy and the length of a healthy life. For example, if we cured cancer or heart disease today, what would that mean for the general population's life expectancy tomorrow? Not much because something else would take people down. You may be able to save yourself from a heart attack or colon cancer, but you won't escape another age-related ailment like kidney disease or a stroke.[9]

I agree with the authors of this study that the potential benefits of slowing aging processes have been underrecognized by most of the scientific community. It's time for an attack on aging itself. To that end, I hope that the Water Principle becomes a much-embraced strategy in that arsenal. It offers a new paradigm of health promotion and disease prevention that could result in longer, more satisfying lives. Because it doesn't focus on just a single disease or condition, it stands to have a much greater impact on the health and wellness of people who take its tenets to heart.

While it's common knowledge that with aging comes disease, few people stop to think about what happens when you reduce aging: you reduce disease. Not only do you reduce the risk factors for disease, but you can even reduce the likelihood that a certain disease will have a maximal effect on you. In other words, when you equip your body with what it needs to function optimally at the cellular level, you effectively shield yourself from age-related diseases, forcing your body to live younger for as long as it can.

» The Three Fountains of Youth

Keeping your vital waters in your cells is the whole point of the Water Principle, but as I've said, this has very little to do with the water you drink. True hydration can originate from unlikely sources. Think of a time when you splurged on a facial or got a massage. Chances are you looked and felt better afterward. Have you ever noticed that after a great night's sleep or just a catnap in the afternoon, you looked fresher in the mirror? How about the last time you went on vacation and came back looking younger and feeling more energetic? This brings me to my three fountains of youth, which reflect the three areas on which to focus that embody the Water Principle. Each of these will be addressed in the three-step program outlined in part 2.

Fountain of Youth I: How You Think and Take Care of Your Emotions

Reducing the negative effects of emotions and stress on the body is key to optimal health. This, of course, includes abandoning the strife for perfection. Patients may come to me with specific dermatological problems to solve, but I can't help them effectively without addressing their psychological and social balance in tandem with their skincare. Science is just beginning to uncover the relationship between our physical and psychological health for it's finally well documented that moods and a condition as serious as depression can increase one's risk for stroke.[10] And of all the "prescriptions" I give patients to help them to look and feel better, the hardest one for them to take is to give themselves permission to live a more imperfect, playful life in the pursuit of happiness and total well-being. In the next chapter, we'll explore the concept of cultural stress, which, as I've already I pointed out, is the most pervasive, harmful type of stress around these days.

The Greek philosopher Plato once described necessity as the mother of invention. Through the years, I've witnessed confirmation of this ancient wisdom in the countless scientific discoveries that began with doctors searching for new and more effective ways to meet the needs of their patients. These findings have shaped, and continue to shape, treatment options and educate professionals in every field of medicine and therapeutic care.

Despite the fact that aging is part of the life cycle, as is the continual decline in function of all your body's systems, we are not on a path of decay and deterioration from the day we are born. Much to the contrary, the body is a remarkable machine—continually repairing itself, replacing lost cells and damaged proteins, making new mitochondria and new molecules, and fixing DNA. Every day your body gives birth to new cells and tissue—out of necessity. Ultimately every cell in your body turns over, from skin cells to heart, lung, and liver cells. Different cells turn over at different times, some faster than others. Imagine the work involved behind those scenes and the compromises that must occur when the body lacks the right raw materials needed for it to function at its optimal level. As the body ages, it requires an increased quantity of these raw materials, and the better you are at supplying them, the more successful you will be at slowing down your aging process.

Fountain of Youth II: What You Put in and on Your Body

It's no surprise that proper nutrition is one of the keys to good health, but what's not commonly understood is that you can maximize your body's capacity to heal itself and support production of robust, healthy, hydrated cells through the foods you put in your mouth. Providing your body with the right raw materials allows it to maintain a healthy water balance, stimulate new cell growth, and repair vital structures. In addition to providing nutrition, we support our skin's health; skin, after all, is your largest organ and the first line of defense against assault from pathogens, UV radiation, chemicals, and physical impact. Because it's a visible organ, it's usually the first place we find signs of aging.

Although we tend to think of the skin as a separate organ, not related to anything else, it's connected to every system in the body— from your cardiovascular and digestive systems to your immune, muscular, reproductive, endocrine, lymphatic, nervous, urinary, and skeletal systems. All must work in synergy for total body health. Both heart and skin, for example, rely on blood veins. This helps explain why when you get angry, your heart beats faster and your face reddens. This interconnectedness between the skin and internal body is largely forgotten by people who see the skin as a separate entity. It's a two-way street. When we damage the skin, we damage our insides. Similarly, what we experience inside our bodies could have manifestations on the outside. As a dermatologist, I came to understand this whole-body connectivity early on, leading me to seek more and more solutions to external skin problems by turning inward and including systemic factors in skin health.

Looking at skin provides a window into cellular and connective tissue health throughout your body. The cyclical process of cellular turnover—the complex phenomenon of tissue growth, repair, and breakdown—says a lot about how we age. When we think of aging on the outside, we are really talking about how fast our collagen and elastin—which keep our external skin springy, resilient, and vibrant—deteriorate over time. Once damaged, these fibers lose water and become dry and brittle, leading to wrinkles and sagging. Water, in fact, is lost from every component of the skin, which explains the difference between a twenty-something's dewy complexion and your grandmother's.

Every system in the body is carefully engineered to operate at a certain balance point for optimal performance. The process through which this balance is maintained is called homeostasis. When anything goes awry, the body automatically goes to work to correct it and bring it back to this balance point. This is why you sweat when your body temperature rises. The sweating cools you off, keeping your body temperature at an ideal 98.6 degrees Fahrenheit. If tissue is damaged or injured, your body will innately know that something is out of alignment and attempt to rebuild it from its components. It's adept at rebuilding tissue as long as it has the parts available. Unfortunately, that is not always the case, ultimately resulting in preventable disease and premature aging as damage builds up and goes unrepaired.

You also need to provide amino acids, the building blocks for collagen and elastin, which help keep your blood vessels firm and hold their shape. Briefly, the breakdown of collagen and elastin is responsible for the primary differences in appearance between an old face and a young face. But internally, the aging of the blood vessels and heart, sometimes called arterial aging, can be deadly. It's responsible for so many age-related diseases that either reduce one's quality of life or just cut life short: strokes, heart attacks, memory loss, and a loss of blood and nutrients to critical organs.

Your body requires nutrients to rehydrate its blood vessels and to attract wasted water back to them. My program focuses on giving you what you need for every system in your body to function optimally—from the cellular level up.

Despite what you might think, there are lots of ways to treat the

Your skin, which accounts for 12 to 16 percent of your body's weight, is not just your largest organ but also the most interconnected. Poets call the eyes the windows to the soul, and perhaps they should call the skin the mirror of your heart, lungs, liver, and kidneys. Classic examples of this connection are the yellow tinge the skin takes on when the liver is in trouble, the red face that can indicate heart trouble, and the edema that indicates kidney trouble.

skin that will reverse visible signs of aging and help prevent further decline. These include appropriate topical skincare regimens that you can follow at home, or with the help of an esthetician at a spa, and cosmetic medical services—all of which I'll cover in chapter 5.

Fundamentally, we now know that the key to healthy skin is found at the cellular level and that a youthful outer layer relies on optimizing the condition of your outermost cells, which are constantly under siege by the environment. Healthy skin cells that can function properly and replicate predictably will preserve your health, hold healthy water in, and ultimately slow down the natural aging process. People often forget that skin cells need the same constant supply of water, oxygen, vitamins, and nutrients as every organ and tissue in the body does. Skin also contains connective tissues that thirst for attention, just like the connective tissues found in blood vessels, nerves, joints, tendons, and ligaments.

Fountain of Youth III: The Magic of Movement

The benefits of exercise are well documented, but if I were to ask you what some of those benefits are, chances are you'd list items like lower heart rate, stronger cardiovascular system, higher lung capacity, weight management, and so on. Indeed, the advantages of being fit are plentiful, but here's one no one mentions or even considers: lower levels of cultural stress and, at the cellular level, better hydration. That's right: in the lab we find that people who maintain a regular physical exercise program—even just a simple, minimal routine a few times a week—have a higher cellular water content. They are able to stay hydrated much more easily than a sedentary person. Why? Muscle—not fat—is the ultimate compartment for cellular water. It holds much more water than fat does, which also explains why bioelectrical pulses sent through a body to measure its composition move quickly through people who carry more muscle than fat. Those pulses speed through water and trip on fat. How fast those pulses move determines your fat-to-muscle ratio.

The lesson: the more muscle you have, the better your chance of supporting cellular water. Exercise ultimately fosters hydration; the fitter you are, the less water you need to drink. (By the way, this has nothing to do with "bulking up." When you build lean muscle, you melt away fat and uncover a toned, healthy, and *hydrated* body. No wonder people glow after exercise!) Being physically active will also spill into other aspects of your life that honor the Water Principle. As you shape up, you'll reach for healthier foods and generally feel motivated to pay greater attention to your lifestyle habits. You'll also be able to combat cultural stress.

Although the power of exercise in reducing stress in general is well known, here's something you might not have known: exercise makes your blood circulate more quickly, transporting the stress hormone (and fat-friendly) cortisol to your kidneys and flushing it out of your system. Cortisol encourages your body to store fat—especially dangerous belly fat—which releases fatty acids into your blood, raising cholesterol and insulin levels and paving the way for heart disease and diabetes. This is why several studies have shown that regular exercise can dramatically help control blood sugar and reduce the risk for metabolic disorders like insulin resistance and type 2 diabetes. One study found walking briskly for a half hour every day reduces the risk of developing type 2 diabetes by 30 percent.[11]

The physical benefits of exercise are no doubt a powerful force against the ravages of aging. And on the flip side of the coin, sedentariness is a destructive force. But if you were to ask me about the biggest common denominator of all when it comes to living a vibrant, long life, one that connects all the information I've given you so far, it's this: combatting cultural stress. I've already mentioned and briefly defined this term, but let's get up close and personal with the concept now that you've gained a broad understanding of my healthcare approach and underlying philosophy. It turns out that combatting cultural stress through the lens of the Water Principle is the ultimate key to reversing aging—and looking and feeling great.

» What's Your Living Age?

I covered a lot of territory in this chapter, and you may be wondering how it all fits together. I started by talking broadly about happiness and how, as we get older, we tend to lose that joyful inner zest like that of a child. It becomes harder to keep a positive attitude given life's trials and our exceedingly high expectations of ourselves. The irony is that as we expect more and more from ourselves and strive to be perfect, we simultaneously fail to put ourselves first and really take care of our bodies from the inside out. Stress becomes more of a challenge to manage, and it shows up in clinical conditions ranging from general anxiety disorders to severe depression. And the more stress you suffer, the unhappier you feel and the faster you age. This can be seen generally in one's overall outer appearance as well as deeply inside via molecular and cellular signs that the body isn't working at optimal capacity—it's not, as it were, keeping its youth and "happy genes" turned on.

Then I went on to explain my Water Principle, which is the idea that aging is directly correlated with the loss of cellular water as your cells become unable to hold vital water to perform optimally and to sustain life. When we are young, we naturally have more water in our cells; as we age we have less. Similarly, when we are happy we have more water in our cells; when we are sad we have less. Note the relationship: cellular hydration is the key to health, happiness, and youthfulness.

In my clinical work and laboratory studies, I've found a parallel relationship between people's general contentment and their cellular water content. Happy people have increased cellular water and look and feel much younger than their chronological age (as much as ten years younger). They also are a lot more adept at handling stress, even when it's constant and severe at times. Conversely, those who show signs of advanced aging usually report being dissatisfied with life, unfulfilled, and unhappy. They let every little stress get to them, and they typically experience much more cultural stress than the average person. And when you quantify their cellular water content, they are indeed "dehydrated." Their cells are not retaining water, and therefore are not performing optimally. (Think about it: when you're under acute stress, one of the body's first reactions is to make you sweat; hence the "sweaty palms" saying. Imagine a similar process going on at the cellular level. Granted, cells don't sweat, but when under stress they can most definitely lose the precious water that holds the nutrients they need to thrive.)

There's a reason why happiness can make your skin glow; the connection between our psychological well-being and physical health is powerful. Picture an ebullient, carefree child (who obviously doesn't have a cell phone or an e-mail account yet). She's young, happy, and hydrated. Now picture the opposite, an old, grumpy woman who has no passion for living. She's no doubt lost cellular water through the normal process of aging, but her water loss will be significantly greater than a peer who kept her inner toddler alive and well throughout life.

People who "age well" don't look their age because they don't act their age.

At least twice a week I hear adults in my medical practice complain that their lives are in a rut—that they feel stuck and have lost the drive and fun factor that they once had in their youth. Every day is the same, and even though they may be very active with social media or busy themselves with a lot of work, at the same time they feel isolated and lonely. It's as if their lives have lost meaning. Nothing gets them excited anymore, and their despair and apathy are practically palpable. Little do they know, however, that a solution exists that has nothing to do with pharmaceutical drugs and everything to do with reigniting the playfulness, creativity, and novelty-seeking behavior of a child. And when they make that change, it's as if magic happens. Something literally gets turned on inside as they go from lifeless to lively. From hopelessness to happiness. From aging fast and losing cellular water to aging gracefully and *using* cellular water to promote health. All of this, in turn, feeds a beautiful cycle of wellness. It is what I call my Circle of Life.

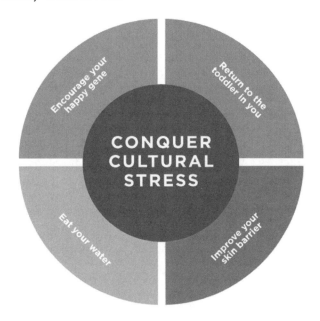

CIRCLE OF LIFE

When new patients go through my program at my health center, I have them first complete an assessment to determine their Living

Age. It's a way of measuring how their current lifestyle is affecting how well they are aging. This is an excellent exercise to do, and below you'll find the same twenty questions my personal patients answer. Answer them all truthfully and score yourself.

This is unlike other health tests you may have taken in the past because it won't ask you about your cholesterol level or number on the scale, so don't panic. Be honest with yourself as you answer these questions; don't try to cheat by giving a "right" answer that you think will boost your score. (i.e., lower your age). There's no one here but you and these responses. The more truthfully you answer these, the better your capacity to transform yourself starting today. Once you've added up the values for all twenty questions, you then add that to your chronological age. So, if the sum of your answers totals -5 and you're forty years old, then your Living Age would be thirty-five years old. Conversely, if your responses amount to +7, then your Living Age would be 47.

A Younger You Assessment

What's Your Living Age?
Use this assessment to determine how you current lifestyle is affecting how well you are aging.

1. When I tell people my real age, they are
   A. amazed—since I look younger
   B. not surprised—since I look as old as I am
   C. trying not to admit I look older than I really am

2. People would describe me as
   A. rigid and set in my ways
   B. someone who sets reasonable boundaries
   C. a pushover

3. I use sunscreen
   A. rarely—since my skin doesn't burn

B. when I plan to be in the sun

C. every day

4. I have _____ close friends (or family members if you have a close relationship)

A. 0–2

B. 3–4

C. 5+

5. Of those friends, I see _____ on a regular basis

A. none of them

B. 1–2 of them

C. all of them

6. I think of manicures, pedicures, and massages as

A. a necessity

B. a luxury

C. something I wish I had time for

7. The most important person in the world is

A. a family member or other loved one

b. me

C. I can't decide

8. I splurge on tasty treats

A. never

B. about 20 percent of the time

C. pretty much whenever I get the chance

9. I exercise

A. rarely—if at all

B. 3–4 times per week; I do something I enjoy like bike riding, gardening, golfing, of dancing

C. 5 or more times each week

10. The last time I did something fun and spontaneous was

A. yesterday

    B. earlier this year

    C. I don't remember

11. I spend _____ of my time in the sun each week

    A. more than 40 percent

    B. 30–40 percent

    C. 20 percent or less

12. When thinking about the next chapter in my life, I am generally

    A. excited and looking forward to whatever life brings

    B. terrified—because I worry about the future

    C. I don't really think about it or care

13. My daily skin treatment consists of

    A. a cleanser, a moisturizer, treatments, and sunscreen

    B. usually just a cleanser and a moisturizer

    C. I don't have a daily skin treatment

14. I check my e-mail

    A. every time it dings

    B. every couple of hours

    C. only during working hours

15. I eat _____ servings of fruits and vegetables each day

    A. 4 or more

    B. 2–3

    C. 0

16. The nutritional supplements I take include

    A. a multivitamin or other supplement

    B. a multivitamin plus additional supplements

    C. I don't take any supplements

17. I eat red meat

    A. very rarely, when I'm craving it

    B. never

    C. pretty much every day

18. I experience stress
    A. chronically—it's never-ending
    B. more times than I'd like to admit
    C. only occasionally

19. When I feel stressed, I
    A. react with anger
    B. retreat within myself
    C. take a deep breath and take it all in

20. I make time for a hobby or do something I love
    A. every day
    B. once a week
    C. I don't know

Your Living Age tells you whether the way you live and the choices you make are adding years to or subtracting years from your real age.

Scoring: In the table below, circle your answer for each question and write the value on the line. Add up the twenty values to calculate your Living Age.

1. A=-1, B=0, C=+1 _____
2. A=0, B=-1, C=+1 _____
3. A=+1, B=0, C=-1 _____
4. A=+1, B=0, C=-1 _____
5. A=+1, B=0, C=-1 _____
6. A=-1, B=+1, C=0 _____
7. A=0, B=-1, C=+1 _____
8. A=0, B=-1, C=+1 _____
9. A=+1, B=0, C=-1 _____
10. A=-1, B=0, C=+1 _____
11. A=+1, B=0, C=-1 _____
12. A=-1, B=+1 C=0 _____
13. A=-1, B=0, C=+1 _____
14. A=+1, B=0, C=-1 _____

15. A=-1, B=0, C=+1 _____
16. A=0, B=-1, C=+1 _____
17. A=0, B=-1, C=+1 _____
18. A=+1, B=0, C=-1 _____
19. A=+1, B=0, C=-1 _____
20. A=-1, B=0, C=+1 _____
YOUR LIVING AGE: _____

» Turning on Your Happy Genes

You can't change the fact that you will age, but by striving to maintain a happy, youthful attitude and youthful levels of cellular hydration, you can actually enjoy the aging process. This theory explains the disparity in apparent age between two people of the same age. The closer a person mirrors the fully hydrated state and happy care-free attitude of a toddler, the younger he or she will look and feel—and truly embracing the inclusive health lifestyle puts you back in touch with the toddler in you. Indeed, you can flip the switch on those happy genes—the genes that relate with increased longevity and psychological well-being. And the key, as you're about to find out, is to conquer cultural stress.

CHAPTER 3

The Modern Scourge: Cultural Stress

Why have a bad day when you can have a good day?

S tress gets a lot of ink in media circles, but one type of stress that's relatively new to us as a people and society is what I call cultural stress—the silent killer. In my opinion, it's among the most pervasive hallmarks of everyday life that can tie a big knot in your attempts to live a healthy life.

While it may seem to be an intangible and invisible behemoth, cultural stress sneakily zooms in on cells and wrings them dry without your necessarily feeling or noticing it at first. Its effects, however, are cumulative and emerge over time. The good news is, managing cultural stress is highly possible, even when regular stress is here to stay.

When was the last time you laughed like a kid? Booked a vacation? Played hooky from work to play with friends in town? Had dinner with someone and truly lost all sense of time and felt really *happy* like the proverbial kid in a candy store?

If you're still thinking about those times, if they even existed, then it has been too long.

My patients inspire me every day. Many of them are suffering way beyond the skin condition that brought them to my examining room. One woman I'll call Jan had psoriasis, which is a crusty and itchy disease that can flare up under stressful situations. When I asked Jan about her daily stress, she confided that her family caused her much stress. She hadn't spoken to her parents for more than a year, she was estranged from her sister, and she was having occasional spats with her husband that disturbed her.

Without even having to perform lab work I knew that her system was depleted. I talked to Jan about her diet, her exercise, and her emotional well-being. I explained that trying to deal with her communication with her family would be an adjunct to the salves and internal treatments I would be prescribing. I also suggested that she might see a psychologist or family therapist to help with those emotional stresses if she couldn't do it alone. Jan was a wonderful listener, and although I was worried that she wouldn't follow my recommendations, she in fact did take me very seriously. Before she returned for her six-week checkup, she called me to relate the story of reconnecting with her sister after talking to a therapist. When she told a similar story about her relationship with her husband, she was so happy that she actually began to cry. Jan realized that she had been so tightly wound up in her problems that she'd forgotten to turn to her husband and simply talk to him.

I share this story because Jan is not alone. It's very easy to forget to communicate with the people we love. It's also very easy to let what I call cultural stress invade our lives. We're busy. We're multitasking. We're commuting. We're obsessively checking our retirement portfolios. We're trying to keep up with ourselves and our racetrack culture at the expense of health and genuine happiness.

In recent studies of the so-called Blue Zones—places where people live long, lean lives well into their nineties and beyond—the common denominator is clear: a low-stress lifestyle.[1] The people in these areas maintain a positive outlook on life, belong to a tightly knit community, and keep family first. They move naturally in everyday life and consume fresh, local ingredients, and processed food is not part of their daily diet. One group in particular—the only one in the United States—is a stone's throw from the densely populated, smoggy city of Los Angeles. This community of Seventh-Day Adventists in Loma Linda, California, defies the stereotype that you have to live like a hermit in a pristine, remote area to avoid a short life. Another group in Sardinia, Italy, comprises sheepherders who spend their days walking, enjoying family and friends routinely, and drinking local red wine with their meals. The famous Okinawan residents of Japan drink mugwort sake, remain active, and honor the elderly. In short, these peoples live by my tenets without even knowing it. Masters of healthy living, they may not even know what stress is, at least not in the same way the average American does.

Emotional care is sorely neglected in our society, yet emotions create a strong and powerful undercurrent to our health. The role of modern medicine is so focused on acute disease that we forget to ask ourselves, "What is true health?"

Not only is the world in which we live causing us to feel time deprived and anxious, but the resultant stress is actually adding tremendous pressure on our biological systems. This is when we sometimes turn to unhealthy habits that push us in the wrong direction and leave us ever-more tired, uncreative, drug and stimulant dependent, and unsatisfied. During the course of my work with more than fifty thousand patients, I've discovered that using the Water Principle to create healthy, hydrated cells helps the body fight aging and disease and, most importantly, the ruinous effects of cultural stress. Since identifying this new type of stress, I've prompted a new field of studies that are now underway to investigate just how influential cultural stress is on health and wellness and what we can do about its negative consequences.

As the world has experienced political, climatological, technological, and cultural changes, a need for a new category of stress is upon us. Cultural stress is man-made, meaning it comes from the evolution of our environment and our reaction to it. However, unlike traditional forms of stress that are critical to survival, it is wholly unnecessary for survival. And it's pervasive, constant, cumulative, superimposing on all other types of stress, and a partner to all other stress types. Cultural stressors are not limited to work, bosses, kids, tardiness, "technostress," and incessant e-mail.

It's not the stress—it is how you respond to it.

Cultural stress is a collection of the daily events ingrained within people's habits because of the perception that these rituals are needed for everyday subsistence. It's also perfectionism that leads to pessimism. Cultural stress is not a discriminatory type of stress as it affects people globally without regard to socioeconomic status, nationality, sex, age, religion, or race. Equally, it can be found not only in the workplace but also at home and in social settings. Because

---

Being truly healthy not only means the body is free of diabetes, cancer, and other afflictions—but also involves a passion for life, a true connection with others, and an overall positive sense of self. If you answer yes to any of the following questions, you are exhibiting symptoms of cultural stress:

- Do you overreact to common irritations—like bad service—with rage or despair?
- Do you fear or dislike changes at work as opportunities and worry about being fired?
- Does 24/7 interactivity have you "logged on" to your job after normal work hours?
- Do you feel anger and anxiety about being late due to everyday traffic congestion?
- Do you lack the time to cook good meals or sleep a full eight hours?

---

of its chronic and pervasive nature, cultural stress may cause many to live in a constant state of resistance and exhaustion. Internally, cultural stress may cause sleep loss and subsequent hormonal instability, increasing the risk for cardiovascular and endocrine diseases. Cultural stress may even indirectly accelerate aging as studies have shown the detrimental effects that can occur to cells and connective tissue. One study shows a direct correlation between sleep loss and telomere shortening.[2]

We are ill adapted to handle this kind of stress, and it could very well be what brings the average life span down for the first time in modern history—rolling back the gains brought by advancements in medicine and technology.

But the good news is, cultural stress is largely manageable. But before we get to those stress antidotes, let's take a look at what stress means and how it affects all of us physically the same, regardless of the specific stressor.

» The Science of Stress

The second you were born was probably the first time your body felt stress, and you probably cried. We've all experienced myriad stressful situations since birth. What stresses you out? Money? Health? Kids? Fear of failure? Perhaps success stresses you out. Ask the question a thousand times and you'll get a thousand different answers. What's clear is that from birth, we live with stress. And today it's become clear that stress is directly linked to the six leading causes of death in the United States, including heart disease, cancer, accidents, and suicide.

Most of us can recognize the symptoms of stress. We feel them. We become irritable, our heart races, our face feels hot, we feel a familiar headache or upset stomach, suddenly our deodorant seems to have lost its power as wetness builds, we experience a feeling of impending doom, and we're irritated by the smallest challenges or mishaps. For some people, stress has little outward effect. For these individuals, what they feel on the surface is internalized and sometimes expressed as depression or disease. In fact, many of these people don't believe they experience stress—but they do. They just don't consciously recognize it until it builds up to a certain point and seeps out in other ways.

The term "stress," as it is used today, was coined by one of the founding fathers of stress research, Hans Selye, in 1936, who defined it as "the non-specific response of the body to any demand for change."[3] Essentially, Selye proposed that when subjected to persistent stress, both humans and animals could develop certain life-threatening afflictions, such as heart attacks and strokes, which were thought to be caused by specific pathogens only. This is a crucial point because it illuminates the impact that everyday life and experiences have not only on our emotional well-being but also on our physical health.

The word "stress" as it relates to emotions became part of our vocabulary in the 1950s.[4] Its use became common with the onset of the Cold War, which was an era when fear ruled. We were frightened of atomic war, so we built bomb shelters. As a society, we could not say we were "afraid"; instead, we used the word "stress." Today, we continue to use the word to describe anything that disrupts us emotionally—we're stressed, stressed out, under stress, and so on. Stress can also be described as the thoughts, feelings, behaviors, and physiological changes that happen when we respond to demands and perceptions. If these demands placed on us overwhelm our perceived ability to cope, we experience stress. We begin to pant silently in our frenzied minds like an animal, probably looking for an escape, too.

Since Selye, researchers have broken stress down into several subcategories. Stress physiology has come a long way particularly in the last fifty years, and so have the stressors. One hundred years ago, people worried about dying from influenza, polio, and giving birth. Now we worry about the illnesses that are likely to creep up on us as we get older and more worn out physically. Those illnesses include the most common killers of today: heart disease, cancer, and stroke. Rather than striking us suddenly like a crouching tiger, these diseases slowly build up over time, gathering strength based on our lifestyles until they finally emerge and either dim our lights or shut them off completely.

Clinically, we now categorize stress in three ways: acute stress, episodic acute stress, and chronic stress.

Acute stress is short term and is the most common form of stress. This type of stress comes from activities like taking a test, giving a speech, or avoiding an accident. Once the test, speech, or threat of an accident is over, the stress goes away. Your body's physical reaction to the stress also wanes, which I'll get to shortly. Acute stress is the most treatable and manageable kind of stress (because it's over pretty quickly!). It's also probably the most ancient form of stress because it's what got us out of life-threatening situations when we were roaming the savannah among wild animals. Millennia ago, threats to our livelihood were more clear cut and we relied on the famous fight-or-flight response to leap out of harm's way. But over the last several hundred years, we've moved out of the real jungle and into a new one of our own making. These days, stress is more likely to come at us from modern aggravations and responsibilities: hearing chronically bad news, driving in commuter traffic, juggling tight finances, and so on. Unlike a brief encounter with a wild animal—an encounter you either win or lose in a matter of seconds—modern stress can often be relentless and the effects are cumulative.

Episodic acute stress happens to those who live in chaos. People who experience this kind of stress seem to always be in a rush, but ironically, they're habitually late. They are supremely busy but don't necessarily get a single task accomplished on time. Or they don't finish projects because they frantically move from one task to another ad nauseam. We all know people who fall into this category.

Chronic stress is often the most debilitating. This is the stress that people feel when they cannot see a way out of a bad situation, and we can find plenty of examples here: an unhappy marriage, an ongoing struggle with a loved one or business partner, a serious health challenge, debt, poverty, a dead-end job, or prolonged unemployment. The economic events of the last decade have led to an epidemic of chronic, unrelenting stress in our world. Those who experience chronic stress tend to lack solid coping skills, and rather than have optimistic outlooks on life no matter what's going on, they ruminate on the past, worry about the future, and generally live with a dark cloud hanging over them. They hold on to their pessimistic attitude like a blanket, despite its harmful effects that are far from comforting.

We are each born with a unique commodity called life. It is stressed by the environment, and it is up to us to make the best of it.

While these three categories were adequate for the last several decades, so much has changed in the years since "stress" first entered our dictionary. It's become necessary to add cultural stress.

» A New Stress Putting Us on the Verge

Cultural stress is a new type of stress that is superimposed on the normal stresses of everyday life. It began infiltrating our lives as we became more technologically savvy and affluent. Technology now allows us to work and communicate anywhere, anytime, twenty-four hours a day, and this makes America the land of the constantly "logged-on" workforce. According to a US government report, Americans work longer hours than nearly anyone in the developed world—even the Japanese.[5] For many professionals, the forty-hour workweek doesn't exist anymore. Sixty- to eighty-hour workweeks are now the norm. We have voice mail, e-mail, texting, and paging and are still bombarded with paper snail mail. From the advent of the

---

Symptoms Associated with Stress*

Cognitive:
- Memory problems
- Inability to concentrate
- Poor judgment
- Pessimistic approach or thoughts
- Anxious or racing thoughts
- Constant worrying

Behavioral symptoms:
- Eating more or less
- Sleeping too much or too little
- Isolating oneself from others
- Procrastinating or neglecting responsibilities
- Using alcohol, cigarettes, or drugs to relax
- Nervous habits (e.g., nail biting, pacing)

Physical symptoms:
- Aches and pains
- Diarrhea or constipation
- Increased frequency of urination
- Indigestion
- Changes in blood glucose
- Nausea, dizziness
- Chest pain, rapid heartbeat
- Loss of sex drive
- Frequent colds
- Irregular periods

Emotional symptoms:
- Moodiness
- Irritability or short temper
- Agitation, inability to relax
- Feeling overwhelmed
- Sense of loneliness and isolation
- Depression or general unhappiness

*Source: Adapted from entries on Wikipedia.com

---

digital revolution in the 1980s to increased population and affluence
to the world-changing events on September 11, 2001, to the recent

climate of unending economic anxiety, many of life's stressors have taken a more prominent and invasive position in our daily lives.

Cultural stress is like a ceaseless refrigerator hum, rather than an infrequent phone ring. Another perfect example of cultural stress is traffic congestion. No matter where you go, it seems that traffic only gets worse. The anxiety, frustration, fear, and reflexes you need to drive defensively, to get from point A to point B on time, add a considerable amount of cultural stress to everyday living. Traffic and driving time must always be considered with our daily schedules, and these thought processes add cultural stress to everything we do. On the other hand, a minor fender-bender is a stand-alone event and an example of basic acute (and sometimes episodic if you experience them on occasion) stress.

Signs of cultural stress are apparent even in infants and young children. One study showed that infants living within one hundred meters of stop-and-go traffic experienced a 2.5-fold increase of non-cold wheezing than those living more than one hundred meters away.[6] These infants experienced constant traffic, noise, and air pollution, which were indicated as prime contributors to the babies' cultural stress levels.

You would think that with all the overworking we do, we'd actually be more productive. To a certain extent, we are. But productivity has its limits. While it's true that stress stimulates a high level of performance, at a certain threshold, performance begins to progressively degrade and negatively affect our output and creativity. It's the classic Law of Diminishing Returns. According to the federal government's National Institute for Occupational Safety and Health, 40 percent of workers find their jobs stressful, and 75 percent of people surveyed believe their jobs are more stressful now than a generation ago.[7] And I think it's quite telling that the World Health Organization has estimated that by the year 2020, depression will be the second leading disability causing disease in the world. In many developed countries, like the United States, depression is already among the top causes in terms of disability and excess mortality.[8]

Here are the top ten sources of cultural stress that I believe impact the average American today:[9]

1. Long commutes: nearly 3.5 million Americans spend an hour and a half or more getting to and from work as they are pushed farther away from work in search of more affordable housing. Rush hours are starting earlier and ending later. Work travel replaces family time.
2. Digital dependence: cell phones, computers, TV—these benefit us in some ways, but because these devices are used 24/7, they tend to lead to information overload.
3. Fear of terrorism.
4. Violent acts of nature.
5. Noise, air, and water pollution (toxicity).
6. Poverty and the high cost of living.
7. Political unrest.
8. Having to keep up with constant new rules and regulations.
9. Overscheduling.
10. The need to achieve, fear of failure, high expectations.

Sadly, cultural stress has taken a huge toll on younger generations, too. It seems like once a week we hear a report in the news about another school shooting, stabbing, or otherwise violent event. I don't think it is a stretch of the imagination to posit that our children are suffering mightily from cultural stress and that today's incidences of bullying, terrorism, and hostility can be attributed to this new stress.

Americans in Isolation

Cultural stress, whether caused by fear, overwork, or too many options causing conflict in decision making, ultimately leads to isolation. I believe isolation to be one of the most prominent diseases in today's world, and new studies are confirming this to be true. New research in mice, for example, suggests that social isolation may promote more damaging inflammation in the brain during a stroke. Researchers found that all the male mice that lived with a female partner survived seven days after a stroke, but only 40 percent of socially isolated animals lived that long.[10] This doesn't mean you have to live with a spouse or partner; you just have to routinely connect with others and stay connected. Studies have also shown that to reduce isolation, people need to have regular physical and social contact, which reduces cultural stress and leads to happier, healthier lives. In my own studies, I've found that the water content of patients who are around others is higher than those who isolate themselves or who don't even realize they isolate themselves until they describe their daily rituals of driving to and from work alone and working in a cubicle all day. This is a modern form of torture. Think about it: what do we do with prisoners who misbehave? We place them in isolation. As highly social, emotional beings, being isolated is distressing.

Isolation can be a self-imposed prison.

And even though we like to think we live in a very connected society now, thanks to e-mail and texting, for example, the very devices we use to communicate can worsen feelings of isolation. We sit and type rather than listen to someone's voice on the phone. We blog about what's going on in our lives to strangers and forget to gather with our nearest and dearest for dinner in person to catch up. There is no substitute for human contact and authentic interactions that don't entail spell checks and links to scripted videos. Real life is never scripted.

Cultural stress starts young. And while parents may not like to hear this, they are the ones who initiate it in their children. New parents are often anxious about getting their child into the best preschool. In fact, it's common for unborn children to be placed on a preschool wait list. The next focus is on ensuring that the child is enrolled in all the right extracurricular activities—from preschool through high school. This cycle puts pressure on children to excel at a very young age, while placing a burden on the parents to make more money to pay for the education and extracurricular activities. No wonder parents are under enormous stress today.

This scenario coupled with our society's increasing financial troubles has a far-reaching domino effect. To make more money to pay for living expenses, we are working longer hours. We are accepting an unprecedented level of stress in our lives. This has put a great strain on our health and well-being, especially because the vast majority of Americans are barely keeping up.

So it's not surprising that over the last few years doctors in all fields of medicine have seen a dramatic change in their patients' stress levels. Patients come into the office with their smart phones and iPads and they tell their physicians how alone they feel, despite the fact that all these communication tools should keep them more connected.

Life is good, bad, and indifferent. Focus on the good.

Anatomy of an Attack

From an evolutionary and survivalist perspective, stress is a good thing. It's supposed to prime the body for battle and get us out of harm's way. The problem, though, is that *our physical reaction is the same every time we sense a potential threat, whether it's real and coming from something truly life-threatening or just a to-do list and an overbearing boss.*

First, the brain signals the adrenal glands to release epinephrine, better known as adrenaline. This is what causes your heart to pick up speed as blood rushes to your muscles in case you need to make a run for it. That adrenaline, by the way, steals blood away from the skin and face to allocate it toward your muscles, which is why you can suddenly look pale as a ghost or become "white with fear."

As soon as the threat passes, your body returns to normal. If the threat doesn't pass and your stress response gets stronger, then a whole wave of stress hormones gets released in a series of events known as the hypothalamic-pituitary-adrenal (HPA) axis. The hypothalamus, a region of the brain, first releases a stress coordinator called corticotropin-releasing hormone (CRH). CRH then delivers a message to a pea-sized gland at the base of your brain called the pituitary, telling it to release another hormone called adrenocorticotropic hormone (ACTH). ACTH then moves through the bloodstream until it hits the adrenals, which then let cortisol loose.

The hypothalamus is frequently referred to as the seat of our emotions. It's our chief leader in emotional processing. The split second you feel anxious, deeply worried, scared, or simply concerned that you can't pay a bill, the hypothalamus secrets CRH, which starts a domino effect ending in cortisol rushing into your bloodstream.

Surely you've heard about cortisol before. It's the body's chief stress hormone, aiding in that famous fight-or-flight response. It also controls how your body processes carbohydrates, fats, and proteins and helps it reduce inflammation. Because it's the hormone responsible for protecting you, its actions increase your appetite and tell your body to stock up on more fat, as well as break down materials, including muscle, that can be used for quick forms of energy. Not at all what you'd like to happen, but when your body senses stress (even when you know it's not the kind that will physically kill you in ten seconds or less), it thinks you won't see food again for a while or it may need an ample supply of fuel to camp out on during a famine or use to make a mad dash. In other words, cortisol causes tissues to break down, including muscle, skin, and collagen, while at the same time it assembles fat.

For this reason, excessive cortisol levels can wreak havoc on the body, making it hard to lose weight, replenish cells, encourage the growth of new cells, and form new youth-building collagen. Everything takes a hit, including blood vessels, which become more fragile and can't keep meeting the demands. As cells lose their capacity to hold onto moisture, they become less resilient. You begin to see this aging on your skin as lines get deeper and more visible on the surface. Imagine what's going on inside. Cellular turnover slows down considerably and you dry out even faster.

Cortisol does, however, serve a positive role. It helps immune cells attack infectious invaders and tells the brain when those invaders have been taken care of. And another way to look at its effects in mobilizing fat and upping your appetite is that it builds up energy reserves (calories) that your muscles may need soon. But for the most part, you don't need those energy reserves because you're not in dire straits. You're just overreacting to a trivial stressor that your body interprets as something serious. And it has a profound impact on you regardless.

Emotional Attachments

I constantly find myself repeating the same message to patients when I explain to them that the skin is connected to their emotions. For centuries, ancient medical practices and cultures have appreciated the connections between mind and body in wellness and disease, yet conventional medicine still trivializes this complex set of relationships. Hopefully that will change given recent evidence.

The scientific study of the impact of stress on the body from the inside out, and even the outside in, has made tremendous advances in the last decade. In 1998, doctors from Harvard University conducted a joint study with several Boston-area hospitals to examine the interactions between the mind and the body through the lens of the skin. They dubbed their findings the NICE (neuro-immuno-cutaneous-endocrine) network. It consists of your nervous system, immune system, the skin, and your endocrine (hormonal) system. All of these are intimately connected through chemicals that transmit messages. It's the body's own personal wireless network, allowing different parts to communicate with each other.[11]

More specifically, these researchers examined how various forces—from aromatherapy and massage to isolation and depression—affect our state of mind and, as a result, overall health and sense of well-being. What they documented confirmed what anecdotal evidence has already implied: our state of mind has a definite impact on our health and even our looks. This helps explain why depressed individuals, for example, look older than they really are and less healthy—not because they've "let themselves go," but because they actually *are* older than happier comrades who are the same biological age. The stress of living with depression has accelerated the aging process and damaged their health.

Another hot area of study in the past decade has been examining the skin's own stress-response system. Research indicated that the skin-centered response has an impact that is on par with the brain-centered HPA axis response. Skin doesn't just respond to the hormonal signals generated by the HPA axis response, even though several hormones and neurotransmitters released inside the body have receptors in the skin. Our skin manages its own independent and fully functional system that acts very much like the HPA axis. It can produce the same molecules locally, including CRH, ACTH, and cortisol. Just as your adrenal glands can release cortisol in a virtual instant, so, too, can pigment cells in your skin and hair follicles release stress hormones.[12]

Skin can also manufacture beta-endorphins, serotonin, and melatonin, the last two of which are hormones key to mood. It's amazing to think our skin has its own stress-response system and shares a common language with our nervous system. Not only does our skin respond to what our brains tell it, but it can initiate responses and send out messages through its own network. This helps explain how myriad psychological and physical (e.g., excessive exposure to the sun's UV rays, a hot stove) stress triggers can have secondary consequences to our appearance and health. Colds become harder to fight, and skin disorders like acne and eczema worsen.

» Cultural Stress and Your Health

Because the body responds to all forms and sources of stress the same, I think cultural stress is having a greater impact on the state of our health than most people realize. (If only our bodies were smart enough to save the stress response for real threats and ignore petty aggravations—we'd be a lot healthier. Maybe in another million years or so.)

In recent years, I have observed an increase in rosacea and adult acne, which I believe are directly related to an increase in cultural stress. Research has already shown that stress can increase the production of certain hormones that worsen acne. One skin condition in particular that I believe may be attributed to cultural stress is an increase in facial hair among adult women, which can be embarrassing to the point of heartbreaking. Nothing is more frustrating than growing hair where it doesn't belong, or where you just don't want it, while losing hair in other places where you *do* want it. Hormonal shifts and the outpouring of androgens, namely testosterone, when you're stressed can cause you to lose hair (e.g., on your head), and it can also cause hair to suddenly appear in places where it didn't previously exist (e.g., on your face and chin).

The good news is, we can counteract cultural stress and improve our health both physically and emotionally with the Water Principle. Cultural stress contributes to damaged cell membranes, which, in turn, allows the precious water that keeps them functioning to escape. The water loss, as you know by now, has myriad effects. It causes our cells and connective tissue to break down, which prevents our heart, lungs, brain, and other organs from functioning at optimal levels—all of which become apparent when you look at the skin. I'm frequently astonished at how much a simple vacation can enhance a patient's health.

Of course, there's more to removing stress from our lives than soaking in a fragrant bath, taking a vacation, or getting a massage. If it were that simple, then many of the stress-induced illnesses and afflictions that we see every day in our world would fade away. The best way to keep stress at bay is to learn how to manage it so it *affects* you less. Toddlers don't stress out the way adults do. So again, tapping that inner toddler can help you out here. And you'll be doing that in part 2.

PART II

YOUR THREE-STEP PLAN

Before commencing my three-step program, your first order of business is to fill out the following questionnaire. I'd like you to come back to this little self-test halfway through your program and then again at the end to check what has improved and what still needs attention.

» Sense of Self Questionnaire

Who is the most important person in your life? (A correct answer to this question exists, and you'll find out about it in chapter 4.) _____

_____

What does your life look like to you? Please rate how satisfied you are with each of the following aspects of your life.

Rank each from 1 to 10. 1 = Not very satisfied, and 10 = Perfectly satisfied

_____ My morning energy is great.

_____ I am at my ideal weight.

_____ I am happy with my appearance.

_____ I love my job and am satisfied by the work (including home-maker, retiree, and volunteer).

_____ I am managing stress successfully.

_____ I am routinely getting as much exercise as I should.

_____ I have a great deal of hope for the future.

_____ My relationships are wonderful and supportive.

_____ My life has the right balance of time for work, relationships, and caring for myself.

_____ Every night I get at least seven to eight hours of uninter-rupted sleep.

CHAPTER 4

Step 1: Let Go of Your Need to Be Perfect

Don't let failure spoil your success.

The headline that ran through the media in 2014 spoke volumes. "Trying to be perfect could be ruining your health: It can trigger heart disease, IBS, and insomnia—and some experts say it could even be as bad for you as smoking," so said *The Daily Mail*.[1] The latest science is pointing to perfectionism as a risk factor for disease in the same way as obesity and using tobacco products.[2] And the latest studies are also revealing that as many as two in five people have perfectionistic tendencies. That's a lot of ill health.

Perfectionism leads to pessimism.

You already know in your heart that taking care of yourself sets the tone for your life and health. You also probably know somewhere deep down that striving for perfection is a setup for failure. Some of us walk around with a keen sense of who we are and what we want to become in life, letting the imperfections be irrelevant. And some of us feel less certain of who we are and continually struggle to find those answers as we try to be perfect. No matter where you are in your own emotional journey, examining your attitude and perspectives is helpful. Finding ways of letting go of perfectionism also helps. How can this be done?

If you take just a few minutes at the end or start of your day to evaluate and write about how you feel and what you're thinking, you can nourish your sense of well-being, peace of mind, and even your capacity to dream big, set realistic goals for the future, and turn imperfections into assets. Self-care begins with self-discovery. And committing your thoughts and ideas to paper can make a huge difference. It provides a record for you while simultaneously offering accountability. It also gives you a chance to adjust your attitude if need be and set a new course that moves you closer to where you want to be.

So few of us take time during the day to turn the volume down on everyone and everything and just sit and think in our own head—in our own creative space and quietude. Following are some questions to help get you started if you don't know what to write about. Use these questions to challenge your view of yourself and as a springboard for self-exploration. There are no wrong or right answers, and no one will be reviewing or judging your responses—so give yourself total freedom. Be honest. Be inspired! Get in touch with your real priorities.

1. What would you do if you knew you could not fail?
2. What job or hobby would you like to try?
3. What can't you live without?
4. What's the one thing you hope to accomplish in your lifetime that you haven't yet?
5. What was your childhood ambition? What is your adult ambition?
6. What's something people might be surprised to learn about you?
7. If you could be anywhere right now, where would you be?
8. Without thinking, name something that makes you happy.

9. What are the top three tasks on your to-do list (that don't entail regular chores and the usual suspects of daily life)?
10. What in life is causing you a great deal of stress and anxiety? How can you begin to remedy that one step at a time?
11. What are you most proud of?
12. If you did not know your age, how old would you want to be?

Feel free to keep multiple journals or use one with different sections to chronicle various aspects and areas in your life. Have one that you use to write down your short-term to-dos. Have another that keeps track of your long-term goals. Yet another journal, a so-called worry journal that houses your concerns, can be very handy for people who have a hard time getting to sleep at night as stressful thoughts intrude and steal much-needed rest time. A worry journal by your bedside can act as a mental depository of your anxieties. Once you write them down, you close the book and tell yourself that you will deal with them tomorrow. Sometimes, you'll find that the act of writing down a worry will lead to solutions that you never thought of before. And this exercise will subconsciously give you hope for your future.

> **An Affirmation a Day**
>
> In appendix A, you'll find 365 insights. That's enough for one a day for an entire year (I've also sprinkled some throughout the book if you haven't noticed). I encourage you to pick one out each day or find one that speaks especially to you and highlight that concept for an entire week. I often have my patients choose one by asking them, "Which one suits you today?"

Last but certainly not least, keep an "On a Positive Note" journal that tracks all the good accomplishments. At the end of the day, even the most stressful of days, stop and reflect: what actually went right? What are you grateful for? What good came out of the day, even if it was unplanned or unexpected? Sometimes, on the worst of days, we can just be thankful that we got through it, and soon we can embrace a whole new day with happy, promising thoughts and intentions.

» The Antidotes to Cultural Stress and the Path to Emotional Youth

I made a huge case for the perils of cultural stress in the previous chapter. The question is, how can you deal with cultural stress without moving to another planet? You are, after all, an adult who has to shoulder the weight of adult realities and stressors to some degree no matter what. As much as we'd like to temporarily return to our toddler years, when we could be freer under the care of someone else, we can't actually do that.

For starters, being fully educated on the different types of stress and their particular effect on you will help you take that initial step in managing stress better. We're living in one of the most exciting times. So much good has come with all the technology and advances we've experienced. Scientifically, we're only just realizing the power of human emotion and its effects on all the body's systems, how it influences skin conditions, and its ability to magnify disease. It's easy to tell people to relax or to be good to themselves, but when stress is so pervasive that no one can hide from or avoid it, it takes effort to unplug.

The reality is that our lives will become even more digitized as time goes on, and we will continue to push our children and ourselves to capacity until we wear out. As Americans, it's not easy to unlearn the need to be on the go, but when it comes to mental and physical health, a day, week, or month of complete relaxation may be just what the doctor ordered. Everything in moderation is the key, and this includes the things that contribute to cultural stress. The goal is to reduce cultural stress while enjoying the simple pleasures of life.

To that end, let me share some ideas to combat cultural stress.

Work with Your Passions, Talents, and Hobbies as Much as Possible

Remember how exciting that first day of school was back when you were in middle school? It's thrilling to enter a new environment, meet new people, and learn something different. Adults trying to keep up with their everyday obligations rarely give themselves permission to act like a schoolgirl or schoolboy again, but doing so can actually have some surprising benefits. In addition to expanding your horizons and exposing you to a new hobby or skill, trying something new can take you just far enough away from your established and routine commitments to give you the feeling that you're on vacation, that you're allowed to goof off and replenish the kid in you who's unencumbered by the banalities of everyday life.

Think of your life as a vacation.

The old phrase "get a life!" has some substance to it. Pursuing a hobby forces you to take time out for yourself and do something enjoyable while providing time for you to reflect. Life seems more worthwhile and pleasurable. And you have reason to seek out others who share your enthusiasm for that hobby, opening the door to connect and relate more with others.

So think about your current hobbies or one you'd like to try and see if you can find a club, group, or class nearby in which to participate. This can include a cooking class, a writing class, a pottery workshop, a photo club, a book club, or, in my case, an art class. And if you can't find anything attuned to your interests, then start your own club or group and invite your friends.

Not all of us can say we are 100 percent satisfied with our current jobs. While time, patience, and trial and error may be needed to find and flourish in a career that's deeply fulfilling and enriching, that doesn't mean you can't find a certain level of enjoyment and gratification in whatever job helps you meet your obligations now. You can continue to explore opportunities in the hopes of finding and establishing yourself in the ideal work scenario. After all, any job is bound to have periods of frustration, high stress, and maybe anguish. Even people who are lucky to have already found their dream job experience challenges that require them to refocus or test a new and unplanned path. Taking stock of your feelings about your work life is critical to taking control of cultural stress; your emotional health is a big piece of the health puzzle. We spend most of our days working, so it's vital that those long days are contributing to our mental and physical health—not taking away from it. This is possible when we strive to align our goals and values with our talents and passions in a job that supports our livelihood and allows us to feel appreciated and needed in the world at large.

Opportunities abound. Keep your eyes open for them.

Get Connected

In search of that holy grail of well-being, many people overlook a powerful weapon that could help them fight illness and depression, speed recovery, slow aging, and prolong life: their friends. We're finally only starting to appreciate the importance of friendship and social networks in overall health. A ten-year Australian study found that older people with a large circle of friends were 22 percent less likely to die during the study period than those with fewer friends.[3] Other studies have further shown that loneliness can be deadlier than the impact of poverty. In the elderly in particular, loneliness has been found to be linked to a 14 percent higher risk of premature death; it's also associated with higher levels of the stress hormone cortisol, which ups one's risk of cardiovascular disease and stroke among other ailments.[4] A large 2007 study published in the prestigious *New*

England Journal of Medicine showed that people whose friends gained weight had a nearly 60 percent increased risk for obesity.[5] And in 2008, Harvard researchers reported that strong social ties could promote brain health as we age.[6] Moreover, new science shows that apathy can signal brain shrinkage, regardless of signs of depression or dementia.[7]

One of the easiest ways to reduce your isolation is to join a group that shares similar hobbies, philosophies, and interests. Some ideas: join a group exercise class or a professional association in your industry, host potluck dinner nights with friends, participate in charity events at your children's schools, or sign up for a class at the nearest community college. Opportunities abound in this department if you open yourself up to them.

> **What can lead to isolation?**
> - Telemedicine
> - Tele-education
> - Teleshopping
> - Teledating
> - Tele-exercising

Disconnect Once in a While

Being attached to machines that allow us to connect with others around the world in an instant has a strange duality. From cell phones to social networks that can transmit what you're doing right now in fractions of a second, communication these days is quick, easy, and to a large degree, isolating. When you resort to electronic transmissions of information rather than speaking to someone in person or even over the phone, you lose the human touch to the experience. You also have a tendency to lose focus as those transmissions become rapid-fire, frequent, distracting, and intrusive. I admire people who make a choice to carve out time once or twice a week when they put down their smart phones and don't check e-mail. Disconnecting yourself occasionally from the digital world can be incredibly invigorating and stress reducing. See if you can designate a single day a week, perhaps a whole weekend from time to time, when you let the voice mail and e-mail pile up. Detach yourself from the need to keep checking and responding to the constant, chattering influx—much of which is not important, not urgent, and not helpful to your health and well-being.

One of the quickest ways to disconnect, even during the middle of a busy workday, is to breathe deeply. Slow, controlled breathing is the foundation for many Eastern practices that aim to immerse the body and mind into a stress-free state. Deep breathing is effective because it causes the parasympathetic nervous system to respond rather than the sympathetic nervous system, which is sensitive to stress and anxiety and is largely responsible for those oft-damaging spikes in the stress hormones cortisol and adrenaline. The response from the parasympathetic nervous system is what leads to a relaxation response characterized by a lower heart rate, relaxed muscles, and reduced blood pressure. And it turns out that deep breathing is a relatively rapid means of getting these two systems to communicate whereby the switch gets flipped from the sympathetic to the parasympathetic.

Deep breathing requires no machines or special location. All you need is a quiet, restful place to sit and close your eyes. Then simply inhale through your nose for as long as you can as your belly rises and the air reaches the top of your lungs. Follow that with a slow exhalation, pushing every bit of breath from your lungs. Continue for at least five rounds of deep breaths.

The benefits of yoga and meditation just rang louder and clearer when a large 2012 report published in the *North American Journal of Medical Science* revealed that the medical literature is filled with proof that these practices confer considerable health benefits, including improved cognition and respiration and reduced cardiovascular risk, body mass index, blood pressure, and diabetes.[8] Yoga also influenced immunity and ameliorated joint disorders. And plenty of studies have shown the power of these practices over stress and depression; one 2013 study in particular highlighted how meditation alone can actually combat stress-induced cellular aging.[9]

Put Yourself First and Splurge Often

Remember the question I asked you on page 78 about who the most important person in your life is?

The answer: you. Indeed, you're more important than anyone else, God included. Now that may seem like an excessively bold statement to make, but consider this: if you don't think you're the most important person in the world, then how can you take care of yourself so that you can show up for everyone else, including your vision of a higher being? You can't. Seeing yourself as "the most important person" isn't about being selfish and egotistical. Far from it. It's the perspective through which you can become the best person you can be and participate in the world in unimaginable ways. It's also the viewpoint through which you can achieve optimal health and happiness.

In the spirit of putting yourself first and combatting cultural stress, I think everyone should visit a spa or massage therapy center as frequently as possible. I know that for many it may seem like a luxury, but it doesn't have to be. If you were to add up the cost of eating dinner out once a week for a month, you'd have yourself plenty of money to get a massage, body scrub, or facial and enjoy the other amenities offered at a spa. Instead of eating out, cook a homemade meal and invite friends over for dinner once a week. Put those extra dollars and toward a monthly or bimonthly spa treatment. The healing power of touch is very real, but very underutilized. I believe that it can be one of the most effective tools for emotional care. Massage not only benefits muscles but also can lower stress levels significantly. Clinical studies show that it can increase weight gain in premature babies, reduce pain in cancer patients, enhance sleep quality, relieve depression, and positively support the immune system.[10] Studies at the renowned Touch Research Institute show that touching is as beneficial as being touched.[11] Scientists are currently figuring out how the body responds to pleasurable touch. So far, we know that a certain class of nerve fibers in the skin called C-tactile nerves are responsible for sending feel-good messages to the brain in response to touch.

Healing touch therapy can take many forms, not just classic massage. Experiment with what your local spa has to offer. Bring this concept home and into the bedroom with your partner, too. In between the more elaborate spa visits, schedule brief, inexpensive manicures or pedicures, or simply exchange five-minute chair massage sessions with your best friend at work. Studies have shown that the latter can dramatically reduce job stress while increasing productivity and alertness.[12]

> *Your harshest critics are really very critical of themselves— not you.*

Give a Little Bit

Regularly plan events with friends and family—people with whom you share deep connections. Setting aside time with those who can help us relax and move away from the limelight of stress is important for not just our emotional health but our physical health, too. Of the patients I've seen who appear to have a tremendous amount of cultural stress in their lives, those who don't have a solid group of friends and regular plans to visit with them are the worst off. Their lab reports and physical exams show signs of accelerated aging. But sometimes, suggesting that they spend more time with friends is not enough. They need to go a step further and engage in an activity that rewards them not just with friendships but with a positive outcome that has the added benefit of helping others. In other words, they need to give back.

Have you ever signed up to volunteer for community events? Have you ever offered your time and expertise to a local youth club, Red Cross chapter, hospital, YMCA chapter, or adult-education center? Have you ever joined a mentorship program that matches you with another individual who wants to learn your skills? Have you ever watched a group of volunteers cleaning up a park or beach and wished you could join them? You can give back in dozens of ways. Though the media likes to focus on how giving back is a practical way in which each one of us can have an impact in the world and effect global change, I like to think about what it gives the person who is doing the giving back: a chance to forge new friendships, to squelch feelings of isolation and stress, and to enjoy the act of making a difference that will surely make a difference on a much smaller—yes, *cellular*—level.

Relax

It sounds almost cliché to say "relax because it will reduce stress" since this is like telling someone not to breathe (or check e-mail). Stress will always be a part of our lives—and our livelihoods. The key is to keep certain sources of unnecessary stress at bay so they don't affect us like a charging rhino. Easier said than done, but here are some ideas to think about this week:

- Can you set a time each day after which you turn off your cell phone and don't respond to nonemergency calls, e-mails, text messages, and so on?
- Can you create a bedtime routine that prepares you for sleep thirty minutes prior to lights out?
- Can you make it a goal to treat yourself once a month or as often as feasible to a massage or another therapeutic treatment of your choice?
- Can you plan your days better so you're not as harried?
- Can you take a recess for some deep breathing or meditation when problems present themselves and your mind starts to race? Problems can easily swell into unmanageable portion sizes for our consciousness and bring us down. They then get out of control and look worse than they really are. Remember, deep breathing or meditation

will help you to gain perspective and reclaim your sanity again.

- Can you get outside more to enjoy the calming effects that only nature can provide? So few of us spend time outdoors anymore. We live and work indoors, often tethered to electronics, meetings, and chores. But it's true that being outdoors and among plants and other living creatures can enhance feelings of health and well-being. This is partly why going for walks and hikes, sailing, skiing, cycling—doing anything in the open air—can be so invigorating. Don't forget to bring the outdoors in, too. Park a big live plant in the room where you spend the most time each day. Set up a reading chair beside a window where you can observe trees and birds.

- Can you pick just a single habit you want to change and commit to making that happen? It can be an ambitious goal like quitting smoking or a small one like reducing your consumption of fast food or replacing butter with extra-virgin olive oil in your cooking.

I know your answer to all these questions is a resounding yes. And if not, then choose to say yes and watch what happens. You'll feel your stress level deflate, and your need to be perfect will vanish.

CHAPTER 5

Step 2: Improve Your Health at a Fundamental Level

Make inclusive health your destiny.

What do scientists look for when they study other planets? Water. Because where there's water, there's *life*. The Water Principle is so simple but so profound: when our cells are not fully hydrated, they deteriorate and cannot function at their peak level. This leads to the tissue damage we refer to as aging. And while this deterioration of the cells ultimately leads to death, before death comes disease, pain, and signs of aging such as wrinkles, inflexibility, fatigue, and loss of mental clarity. Put another way: as we age, we naturally lose water and this water loss, as you know by now, makes it harder for our bodies to heal, scavenge for free radicals, defend against invading bacteria and pathogens, and keep the effects of hormonal imbalance in check. But here's the catch: you can't just drink up to replenish your healing waters. To improve your health at this fundamental level you have to take three chief steps:

- Eat your water
- Feed your face
- Savor sleep

» Eat Your Water, Don't Drink It

Many people wrongly believe that drinking eight, ten, or more glasses of water a day is the answer to health and hydration. The Water Principle is not just about drinking water; it's about getting water *into* the cells and connective tissue and keeping it there so that every cell can function at its full capacity. If we want to make cell membranes stronger, encourage connective tissue regeneration (and hydration), mitigate free-radical damage, and keep the immune response intact, we have to flood the body with nutrients.

So contrary to popular thought, hydrating the body is not about drinking a certain amount of water each day, and the best source of water is far from glacial-fed streams. In fact, we can drink gallons of premium water a day and never become positively hydrated. If we can't keep the water in our cells, we'll be heading to the bathroom all day long. It passes right through instead of staying in the cells and nurturing the body. That's because the cell membranes are damaged; like a bag with holes in which you're trying to hold coins, the cells themselves cannot properly retain water. The water seeps out of the cells where it belongs and becomes wastewater, the kind that I've already stated shows up as swollen legs and ankles, puffy eyes, and bloating.

I'm not the only one who thinks that the eight-glasses-of-water-a-day rule is a sham. In early 2008, researchers from the Indiana University School of Medicine made a list of common medical beliefs espoused by physicians and the general public, myths that either are totally false or lack scientific evidence to support them. They included statements they had heard endorsed by doctors on multiple occasions. The number one myth listed that has been widely repeated by doctors and in the media, was this: people should drink at least eight glasses of water a day.

The study's authors, Dr. Rachel C. Vreeman and Dr. Aaron E. Carroll, found no scientific evidence for this advice.[1] They did find several unsubstantiated recommendations in the popular press, which no doubt you've heard as well. The original culprit? It seems that a 1945 article from the National Research Council, which is part of the National Academy of Sciences, noted that a "suitable allowance" of water for adults is 2.5 liters a day. The exact statement made (pay attention here!): "A suitable allowance of water for adults is 2.5 liters daily in most instances. An ordinary standard for diverse persons is 1 milliliter for each calorie of food. Most of this quantity is contained in prepared foods."[2]

If you ignore the last part of that comment—*most of this quantity is in foods*—then you may get the impression that you need to drink 2.5 liters of water a day. Not so. It's easy to get the 2.5 liters per day without drinking copious amounts of water. The most prevalent ingredient in fruits and vegetables is water.

That is why the best source of high-quality water is at your local farmer's market or grocery store that stocks plenty of fresh produce. The mantra spoken at my Inclusive Health Center is "eat your water—don't drink it." Virtually all food has some water in it, but the most natural whole foods have the highest water content, as well as an abundance of health-promoting ingredients only Mother Nature can provide. Colorful fruits and vegetables, which contain 85 to 98 percent water, concentrate nutrients in their water, thus making it structured—the best form of water for your cells because it stays in your system long enough for your body to put it to good use. Watermelon, for example, is 97 percent water, cucumbers are 97 percent water, tomatoes and zucchini are 95 percent, eggplant is 92 percent, carrots are 88 percent, and peaches are 87 percent water. Foods you'd call dry can also be great sources of water. One slice of whole-wheat bread is about one-third water and a tortilla somewhat more. A roasted chicken breast is 65 percent water, baked salmon is 62 percent, and cheeses like blue and cheddar are about 40 percent water. Beans, grains, and pasta act like sponges when you cook them, which is why a cup of red kidney beans is 77 percent water and couscous is 50 percent water. (Caveat: boiling vegetables leads to water loss because the heat breaks down the cell membranes and allows some of the water to leak out of the cells. For this reason, vegetables weigh less after boiling in water than they did before, which is why I recommend eating as many raw vegetables as possible.)

The advice to eat more fruits and vegetables has been around for a long time, but unfortunately it's not well followed. In 2009, a study out of Queen's University in Ontario, Canada, looked at the fruit and vegetable consumption of nearly two hundred thousand people in developing countries and found that most people don't get their fill.[3] Overall, 77.6 percent of men and 78.4 percent of women consumed less than the suggested five daily servings of produce. The Canadian researchers, who published their findings in the *American Journal of Preventive Medicine*, also noted that low fruit and vegetable consumption is a risk factor for being overweight and obese, while adequate consumption decreases the risk for developing several chronic diseases.

According to the U.S. Centers for Disease Control and Prevention, nearly 70 percent of American adults eat fruit less than two times daily and almost 75 percent consume vegetables less than three times per day.[4]

So why are we having such a hard time eating more fruits and vegetables? It's a question of lifestyle. On the one hand, we are bombarded by processed foods and seduced by their convenience. On the other hand, some of us have been wrongly taught that fruit can cause weight gain due to its sugar content and that starchy vegetables like squash and potatoes are "bad" because they contain so many carbohydrates. Much to the contrary, fruits and vegetables contain a wealth of nutrients that support cellular health and facilitate the transportation of water into the cells for use. Have you ever seen an obese person who says the bulk of his or her diet is composed of natural fruits and vegetables? The complex carbohydrates found in vegetables like squash and potatoes actually feed your brain and your muscles and even fuel your metabolism (and hence, your ability to maintain—or lose—weight). And nothing is more quick and convenient than fresh produce, which is widely available to most of us with very little effort.

We tend to think of food in terms of calories and fat. If you had to rank a list of foods from top to bottom, the unhealthiest being at the bottom, you wouldn't have a problem putting tomatoes near the top and cookies near the bottom. But I want you to try to begin to see foods in terms of how *hydrating* they are, not whether they are "good" or "bad." Under this perspective, tomatoes would still rank high, and items like cookies, chips, pastries, and high-fat and high-sugar foods would rank near the bottom. These bottom dwellers are low in water and can actually be dehydrating. When we consume foods that contain high levels of water, our bodies don't have to expend precious water to digest and process them. The water we eat goes toward replenishing our cellular water and maintaining optimal cellular functions.

Here's another way to look at it. Sugar, salt, and unhealthy fat—the top ingredients in foods we typically overconsume—have virtually no water in them at all. And while we do need salt for survival, it can be very dehydrating and toxic to the body when overconsumed. Processed and fast foods contain large amounts of salt. For the most part, restaurant foods are also high in sodium, especially soups and sauces.

One more point about fruits and vegetables: they contain an ingredient that can help flush excess calories out of the body naturally, reduce your risk for a medley of diseases, curb your appetite, lower your cholesterol, stabilize your blood sugars, improve your immunity, streamline your digestion, and keep you regular. It's called fiber, and it's been a popular subject in research circles lately because of all the positive benefits now associated with fiber. It not only helps one maintain an ideal weight but can prevent cancer. When patients complain about a slow digestion, I tell them to eat more fiber. Digestion slows with age, and fiber helps keep it up to speed.

Technically, fiber is the part of a food that cannot be digested or broken down into a form of energy for the body. This is why it has no calories and isn't really a nutrient. It's considered a type of carbohydrate, but it cannot be absorbed to produce energy. Animal products do not contain fiber—it's found only in a plant's cell walls, which is why it comes from fruits, vegetables, nuts, grains, and seeds. Put simply, fiber is a part of energy-rich, antioxidant-rich, and disease-preventing foods.

You might be wondering how fiber manages to grab on to calories and sweep them out of your system. The mechanism is actually quite simple. Fiber works in the intestines to block the absorption of some of the calories from carbohydrates and fats. Think of fiber as an escort that leads calories out of the body. But does this mean that fiber also grabs on to good nutrients and vitamins? Fortunately, there's been no evidence that fiber simultaneously prevents your body's ability to retain the nutrients it needs. In fact, the reverse has been shown: fiber can enhance your body's absorption of nutrients.

Water-rich foods comprise the best diet plan.

In the last century, we've gone from getting plenty of fiber in our diets to having very little. In the early 1900s, the processing and packaging of food became an enormous growth industry, "freeing" us from the need to grow our food, to eat food seasonally, and to replenish items that could not be stored. Almost overnight, we went from eating fresh foods to eating designer foods loaded with sugar, fat, and salt. And almost overnight, our rates of obesity and diseases such as heart disease, diabetes, and cancer skyrocketed. Today, food processing is the largest industry in the world and, unfortunately, an industry that processes a lot of fiber and other key nutrients *out* of our diet. Meanwhile, it has managed to pack a lot of ingredients into our diet that can actually hijack our brains and compel us to eat more and more of the foods that bankrupt our cells. And it doesn't help that the industry's marketing ploys are quite enticing and convincing.

Fortunately, you can choose to make good decisions when it comes to rediscovering nutrition and fiber in your food, and you don't have to give up delicious taste to do so. Most people would do well to get at least 30 to 35 grams of fiber a day. This can be hard to accomplish if processed food is the norm or if animal products outpace fruits, vegetables, and whole grains in your diet. If you follow my Pitcher of Health, however, you'll be sure to get plenty of fiber.

Three Secrets to Getting More Fiber

- Fill up in the morning: Start the day with a high-fiber breakfast. A bowl of steel-cut oatmeal with a tablespoon or two of flaxseed meal can pack a powerful punch of fiber. Add to that some blueberries, half a banana, and a few crushed walnuts and you'll be set for hours.
- Read labels: A food label can say it's a "good source" of fiber if it contributes 10 percent of your daily value of fiber, which is only about 2.5 grams because the current daily value is low (25 grams). A label can claim a food is "rich in," "high in," or an "excellent source of" fiber if it provides 5 grams of fiber per serving. Some whole-grain cereals are high in fiber.
- Eat the skins of fruits and vegetables, but choose organic: The skins of apples, peaches, potatoes, and zucchini, for example, contain the lion's share of the fiber, so don't peel them off. But do eat organic since you don't want to also consume residue from pesticides often found on the skins.

The Pitcher of Health

The average American is exposed to thousands of calories a day through television, radio, and print ads. Brain researchers increasingly report that fat-and-sugar combinations in particular light up the brain's dopamine pathway, which is a pleasure-sensing spot implicated in people's addictions to alcohol or drugs. The more we see food, the more we want to eat it. Just thinking about a food increases your likelihood that you'll eat it. The good news: that's also true of healthy foods. So looking at a delicious salad or thinking how you'll feel after you eat it may be enough to take your mind off some chain restaurant's advertisement for a bottomless bowl of bread.

In recent years we've heard a lot of noise about the value of eating organic, whole, and "healthy" foods and that low-fat, "good-carb" diets are best. But the truth remains that you could still be missing the mark when it comes to getting the necessary nutrients. How many people do you know who have gone on traditional diets by restricting and eliminating certain foods, opted for "healthy" alternatives, yet still had trouble losing weight? Although this is not a diet book, you will lose weight if you follow my nutritional recommendations. Remember the goal: to put water back into your cells and keep it there. To accomplish this, you need to make sure your body is flooded with nutrients that will strengthen cell membranes and connective tissue so they hold in the good water. This water will help you maximize and even accelerate your metabolism, sculpt stronger muscles, lift your mood, burn unwanted fat, and essentially live young. In doing so, you'll give your body what it needs to heal itself and prevent the onset of disease.

Although new studies show that Americans are trying to eat healthier by cutting calories and eating out less, the majority of us are overweight or obese—and chronically dehydrated.[5] What if we've been focusing on the wrong thing? What if, instead of thinking about limiting grams of fat or which carbs to avoid, we simply ate the foods that feed our cellular membranes and encourage healthy cellular water? I think we'd see a change, and all the problems about weight would take care of themselves. Correction: I *know* we'd see a change because I've watched hundreds of my own patients do just that.

The problem with most diets (even ones where you're simply trying to eat better regardless of weight) is that they tell you what *not* to eat, which often deprives you of critical nutrients *and* your emotional stability. Thanks to the media and recent diet books, you understand now that trans fat, refined sugar, sodium, and processed and classic fast food should be regulated in your diet. You don't need another book to tell you that. But I find that people forget to consider what they could be *missing* in their wholehearted attempts to shape up and trim down. And yes, what you could be missing probably includes healthy sugars and healthy fats. Nothing is more dehydrating than going on a nonfat, low-carb diet taken to the extreme.

It's really true that we are what we eat. If you performed a complete chemical analysis of your body, the report would list materials similar to those found in foods: fat molecules, carbohydrates, protein complexes, and vitamins and minerals that help you to metabolize food and generate the energy you need to live. Think of the body as a self-maintaining factory; it is constantly regenerating itself down to every cell. Each month our skin renews, and about every five days we have a new stomach lining. To renew and rebuild these organs and tissues, our bodies need to be supplied with the elements that have been lost as a result of constant use, degeneration, or aging.

All things considered, it is important to understand that for most people, it's not about what they do or don't eat or drink, it's about the fact that they are unable to keep the water they consume within their cells' membranes. And they can do this only with an adequate supply of five essential ingredients: (1) amino acids, which are the building blocks of proteins; (2) glucosamines, which are amino sugars that build connective tissue; (3) essential fatty acids; (4) lecithin (described below), which contains a key ingredient in cell membranes; and (5) antioxidants.

With the appropriate amount of these nutrients, which are sorely lacking in the standard American diet, the body can maintain and build healthy, strong cell membranes that are critical to keep water from leaking out. That's exactly what the diet recommendations here will help you achieve. And let me tell you, these nutrients come in the most delicious foods ever made on earth. This is the un-diet. You won't have to become vegan or quit your normal dietary habits cold turkey. All I ask is that you do your best to add my recommendations to your life and watch what happens. *Feel* what happens!

At my health center, we don't use food pyramids or plates to teach lessons on how to eat. A few years ago I created my Pitcher of Health to convey optimal eating principles. And consider the symbolism of a pitcher—a vessel that provides water. The food groups within the pitcher encourage intracellular water as they give the body the nutrients it needs to feed cells for overall health. It's designed to help you make the best food choices to consume the optimum level of nutrients necessary for slowing or reversing age-related cellular deterioration and improving cellular water. Highlighting fruits and vegetables above all other foods, it's a road map to maximum rejuvenation internally, externally, *and emotionally.* The food-mood connection is powerful, and anyone who has ever overeaten or rushed to the kitchen during times of stress and anxiety knows what I mean. Mood-driven trips to the pantry or refrigerator, however, can result in reaching for foods that will drain your cells and deepen your dehydration.

As you can see, fruits and vegetables form the base of the pitcher. These are your best sources of water, fiber, and a huge range of macro- and micronutrients, including phytochemicals that are nature's most powerful antioxidants. These foods should make up the bulk of your diet. That is, we should eat more of these foods than those from any other group—three or more servings a day of fruits and five or more servings of vegetables—for example, a small or medium-sized fruit like an apple is one serving and a half cup of chopped vegetable is one serving. This is no joke: a study from the National Bureau of Economic Research found that people who eat at least seven servings of fruits and vegetables each day are happier than those who eat very few fruits and vegetables.[6] Below you'll find lists of my favorite fruits and vegetables.

Whole grains (four to eight servings daily) form the next level up in the pitcher. These are your best sources of the complex carbohydrates that give you long-lasting energy, and they are treasure troves of fiber, minerals, and vitamins. In particular, whole grains are sources of magnesium and selenium, and their shell may act like glucosamine to help build collagen. Magnesium is a mineral used in building bones and releasing energy from muscles. Selenium protects cells from oxidation, and it is also important for a healthy immune system. Glucosamine is necessary for building collagen and connective tissue that is continually breaking down as you age. A serving would be one slice of whole-grain bread or a third cup of cooked brown rice. Avoid refined grains and carbohydrates (sugars).

Proteins (four to six servings daily) is the third level up inside the pitcher. They include omega-3-rich fish, white-meat chicken, eggs, soy foods, fat-free and low-fat dairy products, and beans. Proteins provide most of the amino acids we need for the cellular renewal that keeps all our organs and systems functioning at an optimal level. A serving would be one medium egg or three ounces of fish. Avoid high-saturated-fat meat products and whole-fat dairy foods.

Healthy fats should be limited to just three to four servings a day and are next up within the pitcher. All fats are not created equal. The foods featured are great sources of the omega fats that moderate cholesterol, support nerve function, and help your body build strong cells that attract and retain water. Wonderful as they are, even good fats need to be consumed sparingly because they are so energy-dense that they can be fattening if consumed in excess. One serving would be a teaspoon of olive oil or six almonds. "Healthy" fats are unsaturated, such as omega-3, -6, and -9 fatty acids, which are found in flaxseed oil, extra-virgin olive oil, canola oil, natural-style nut butters, cold-water fish, and nuts. (More on healthy fats coming up.)

Near the top of the pitcher is space for supplements and water to address any dietary deficiencies. Whether or not you choose to take vitamins and supplements is up to you. The use of vitamins and supplements has been called into question by new science that shows they may not offer the kind of benefits we thought they did; and some of them, when consumed in excess, could actually be harmful. That said, many of my own patients report feeling better when they take vitamins and supplements so this might be an area to discuss with your physician.

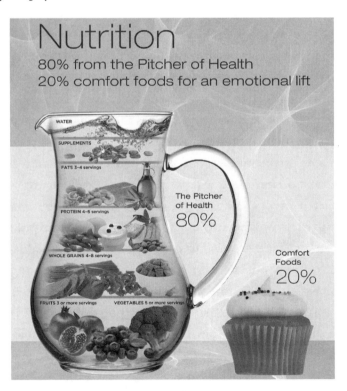

I recommend using the 80/20 rule: eat according to this plan at least 80 percent of the time, and feel free to indulge in a few treats or favorites that aren't mentioned above (like ice cream and cupcakes) no more than 20 percent of the time. Why the 20 percent? If you don't reserve 20 percent for fun foods, you will crave them. It's important to make eating pleasant and the few extra calories from the 20 percent actually reduce the stress of eating. Use the Pitcher as a guide, and choose the foods you

> Before there was medicine, there was food. And before there was food, there was chocolate.

enjoy; don't get stressed out about it. As I said above, approach this diet as one that teaches you how to add the nutrients you're lacking rather than eliminating anything. That slight shift in your thinking can be a powerful motivator.

Water Bombs

Here are my favorite fruits (raw and fresh, unsweetened frozen). Go organic wherever possible, but be sure to *always* buy organic for those marked with an asterisk because they can contain high levels of pesticides when grown conventionally.

Apples*	Goji berries	Papayas
Apricots	Grapefruits	Peaches*
Avocados	Grapes (purple, red,	Pears*
Bananas	green; buy organic if	Pineapples
Blackberries	imported*)	Plums
Black currants	Hawthorn berries	Pomegranates
Blueberries	Honeydew melons	Prunes
Cantaloupes	Kiwis	Raisins
Cherries*	Mangoes	Raspberries
Cranberries	Mulberries	Strawberries*
Elderberries	Nectarines*	Tangerines
Figs	Oranges	Watermelons

Equal parts vegetable and vegging out will keep the doctor away.

Here are my favorite vegetables (raw and fresh, unsweetened frozen, lightly cooked). Again, go organic whenever possible, but be sure to choose organic varieties for those marked with an asterisk.

Artichokes	Eggplant	Pumpkin
Arugula	Garlic	Radishes
Asparagus	Ginger	Seaweed
Beets	Green beans	Shallots
Bok choy	Jicama	Spinach*
Broccoli	Kale	Squash (winter,
Broccoli sprouts	Lettuce*	butternut)
Brussels sprouts	Mustard greens	Sweet potatoes/
Cabbage (green and	Onions (white, red,	yams
red)	and green)	Taro
Carrots	Parsley	Tomatoes
Cauliflower	Parsnips	Turnip greens
Celery*	Peas	Watercress
Collard greens	Peppers* (green,	Wax beans
Corn	yellow, orange, red)	Zucchini
Cucumbers	Potatoes* (white,	
	yellow, red, purple)	

Cleaning out your kitchen and pantry and restocking it with fresh ingredients can be an exhilarating and motivating experience. You may even feel inspired to toss out foods that have been contributing to an unhealthy eating pattern, such as lard, margarine, dry and dehydrating snack foods, low-fiber/high-sugar cereals, refined bread, corn-syrup-driven sauces and condiments, and packaged goods that seem to have an oddly long shelf life.

» Nourish Your Brain with Healthy Fats

There's a reason certain fats are necessary for survival—and sanity. About two-thirds of our brains are composed of fat, and the protective sheath around communicating neurons is 70 percent fat. So in a sense, we need fat to think and to maintain healthy brain function; in particular, the two classes of essential fatty acids called the omega-3s and omega-6s play a crucial role in brain function as well as normal growth and development. This explains why foods like salmon are often called brain food. The omega-3 fats found in salmon, as well as other cold-water fish,

Eat your sunscreen: many of the colorful fruits and vegetables listed contain chemicals that naturally help protect your skin from the harmful effects of UV rays.

avocados, walnuts, flaxseeds, and olives, have numerous proven health benefits, including protecting the heart. Healthy fats are at an all-time low in people's diets, whereas unhealthy fats (e.g., saturated and trans fats) are at an all-time high. But the healthy fats help fat-soluble vitamins such as A, D, E, and K move around the body, create sex hormones, build cell membranes, lower LDL (bad) cholesterol while raising HDL (good) cholesterol, and contribute to the health of skin, eyes, nails, and hair.

In the omega-6 family, gamma linolenic acid (also known as GLA) is one of the all-star anti-inflammatories and soothers. Well known as a stress-reducing nutrient, GLA is largely deficient in the standard American diet because it's a rare oil, found in seed oils such as borage oil, evening primrose oil, black currant oil, and hemp oil.

People are more likely to overdo other omega-6s from sources such as refined vegetable oils, which can actually *increase*—not decrease— inflammation. Soybean oil, for example, is ubiquitous in fast foods and processed foods; in fact, 20 percent of the calories in the American diet are estimated to come from this single source. This can create an imbalance of too many omega-6s and not enough omega-3s, which is partly being blamed for the rise of myriad diseases, from asthma and heart disease to many forms of cancer and autoimmune diseases. The imbalance may also contribute to obesity, depression, dyslexia, and hyperactivity. One now-famous study done in the early 2000s showed that violence in a British prison dropped by 37 percent after omega-3 oils and vitamins were added to the prisoners' diets.[7]

Getting a good balance of these fats is pretty easy. Simply reduce your consumption of processed and fast foods; also reduce the use and consumption of polyunsaturated vegetable oils (e.g., corn, sunflower, safflower, soy, and cottonseed oils). Switch to extra-virgin olive oil as much as possible, even when cooking. Eat more oily fish (salmon, sardines, herring, mackerel, black cod, and bluefish), as well as walnuts, flaxseeds, and omega-3-fortified eggs.

Let Lecithin In

Lecithin is a fatty substance found in all living cells as a major component of cell membranes. It repairs tissues by helping your body build cells with strong, watertight membranes to repair your organs and keep them fully hydrated and functioning at their highest level. It also helps prevent gallstones and improve short-term memory. Ensure you're getting plenty of this cell-hydrating powerhouse by choosing lecithin-rich foods: eggs, non-GMO (genetically modified organism) soy products, cauliflower, peanuts and peanut butter, oranges, potatoes, spinach, iceberg lettuce, and tomatoes.

Eat Up Antioxidants

As I've already hinted at, plants offer the best source of antioxidants—the crusaders against free radicals. Antioxidants will eat up those free radicals, preventing damage and ultimately boosting hydration in cells and tissues. While citrus fruits and berries are sources of the most plentiful antioxidants, all fruits and vegetables provide good supplies of antioxidants. The deeper and brighter the color of the food, the more densely packed with vitamins it is. Buy the most vivid fruits and veggies you can find. Here are the all-stars:

- Blueberries, raspberries, and strawberries
- Pomegranates
- Goji berries
- Vitamin A sources: carrots and mangoes
- Vitamin C sources: kiwis, mangoes, papayas, and black currants
- Vitamin E sources: vegetables oils, almonds, wheat germ, dark green leafy vegetables

Slash the Salt and Spice It Up

Instead of using salt, which can lead to cell damage and retention of extracellular wastewater, try seasoning your meals with these herbs and spices:

- *Ginger*: Ginger is recognized as helpful for motion sickness, migraines, high blood pressure, high cholesterol, arthritis, and blood clots.
- *Turmeric*: Turmeric is currently being studied as a treatment for cancer, Alzheimer's disease, and diabetes, and its anti-inflammatory powers are being evaluated to develop treatments for arthritis.
- *Chili and cayenne*: Capsaicin in chilies thins mucus, and emerging evidence suggests peppers can prevent stomach ulcers and reduce the risk of high blood pressure, stroke, and heart disease.
- *Garlic*: Garlic lowers cholesterol and triglycerides while it thins the blood to help prevent high blood pressure, heart disease, and stroke. Garlic has also been linked to a reduction in the risk of cancers of the stomach and colon.
- *Cumin*: Cumin is a great natural detoxifier. It increases body heat, boosting metabolism and improving kidney

and liver function. Cumin is also a great source of iron, which helps maintain healthy energy levels.

- *Mustard seed*: Mustard seed has been linked to a lower risk of cancer and is a good source of selenium, omega-3 fats, phosphorus, magnesium, manganese, iron, calcium, protein, niacin, and zinc.

Drink as Clean as Possible

I'm not the first to tell you to skip or limit soda pop (diet and regular), sugar-laden fruit juices, and alcohol. Feel free to drink coffee and tea, but be careful to avoid caffeine after two o'clock in the afternoon or you risk having trouble getting a good night's sleep. For many, coffee is the number one source of antioxidants daily, but see if you can get more antioxidants from your fruits and veggies rather than relying on another cup of coffee.

If you choose an alcoholic beverage, red wine is best because it naturally contains antioxidants and minerals. "Moderation" here means one six-ounce glass of wine a day for women and two for men. Have wine with food.

Don't panic if you're still asking, "What do I eat?" I'll give you a week's worth of menu ideas in chapter 7 so you know how to put the Pitcher of Health into action.

» Feed Your Face

It wouldn't surprise me to learn that the vast majority of people don't keep a regular skincare routine. The consequences aren't as painful as, say, not brushing your teeth every day. But they can be very noticeable in the decline of your looks and acceleration of your physical age, which in turn affect your attitude and sense of self. The time it takes to treat your face is the same as it is to brush your teeth—about two minutes. Any drugstore carries the products you need to get started.

Everything you do to meet your daily skincare needs should contain the appropriate ingredients and, above all, be simple and quick. You want to cleanse your skin, treat it with anti-aging products, moisturize it, and protect it with sunscreen. If you have special concerns such as acne, discoloration, and advanced aging, you will need to make some slight modifications.

Here's the 411 on skincare, step by step:

1. *Use a gentle cleanser*: Wash your face twice a day with a gentle cleanser. This will remove dirt, debris, makeup, flakes of dead skin cells, and accumulated oils. Choosing a cleanser is a trial-and-error process. If your face feels dry, taut, and stiff thirty minutes after a wash, the cleanser is too harsh and you should try another one. Your skin should feel soft and pliable a half hour after you wash your face. A cleanser with hydroxy acids such as glycolic and salicylic acids is useful for most people because they exfoliate the skin during the cleansing process and enhance hydration. Depending on your skin type, you may want to use an AHA/BHA (alpha and beta hydroxy acid) skin cleanser every day, twice weekly, or just once a week. If you are prone to acne, then you'll find cleansers designated for acne that contain special ingredients (notably benzoyl peroxide and/or salicylic acid) to help clear bacteria on the skin's surface that can lead to breakouts. Make sure to wash your face with warm—not hot—water. If you find benzoyl peroxide too drying and irritating, then keep to just salicylic acid and be sure to moisturize. Don't be afraid to moisturize skin even though you have acne. It won't worsen it and may, in fact, help treat it.

2. *Apply toner*: Applied to freshly washed skin, toners help return the skin to a slightly acidic pH, where skin

functions best. The protective layer on your skin that helps cripple growing bacteria and fungi while holding moisture in prefers an acidic environment. Most cleansers leave skin slightly on the alkaline (basic) side, which can make you more vulnerable to damage and infection. Even though your skin will naturally go back to a slightly acidic state, toners are refreshing and hydrating and prep the skin for your moisturizer. If you choose to use a toner, make sure it's not too drying (some use harsh alcohols that can dry you out), and ideally find one that contains skin-soothing botanicals, such as mint, cornflower, chamomile, and bitter orange. Some toners also contain hydrating ingredients like sodium pyroglutamic acid (sodium PCA) and amino acids. Those with antioxidants such as vitamins C and E offer an added bonus.

3. *Treat and repair*: If you are using any special formulas, such as retinoids, antioxidant infusions, or solutions for hyperpigmentation, you'd apply those before applying your moisturizer. Follow the instructions that come with the packaging. Some are best used at night or both morning and night.

4. *Moisturize*: Always use a facial moisturizer with sunscreen in the morning. At night, switch to a thicker sunscreen-free formula that is loaded with rich hydrators, antioxidants, and plant extracts. Don't worry about doubling up on ingredients like antioxidants and skin soothers if they are in both your treat-and-repair formulas and your moisturizer. You can't ever get enough of these anti-aging miracles. You may also find a night formula that contains retinols, and that's okay too. If you use a prescription-strength retinoid such as Retin-A, however, skip the night creams with added retinols.

Sometimes I am asked why it's necessary to go through this routine every single day. Well, as I said, it's like brushing your teeth. If you skip a day or two or three, you have lots of buildup to deal with, and you're not likely to get it all in one clean sweep. Wait too long to brush those pearly whites and you're likely to suffer from dental decay and inflamed gums; similarly, you'll see breakouts on your face and clogged pores if you neglect your face. It's not a pretty sight. So feed your face—every single day. (Your teeth, too.)

As for exfoliating, that's a personal choice based on how sensitive your skin is and what you can tolerate. As often as your skin can take it is best. It's the difference between cleaning a floor routinely and hiring a professional cleaning crew after the floor has been left alone too long and becomes a grimy mess. If you use a light exfoliant such as a hydroxy-acid wash, you should be able to exfoliate a few times a week. Go for the heavier-duty exfoliants, such as a facial or microdermabrasion, a few times a year.

You'll want to visit a dermatologist once a year for a routine checkup and to address any specific concerns you have that you cannot seem to solve on your own. However, once you reach your thirties, scheduling visits a few times a year to a trained esthetician (who can be working in a dermatologist's office or a spa) equipped to deliver pharmaceutical-grade treatments can be an excellent part of your wellness plan. Your particular skin needs will determine how frequently you go and which level of treatment you get.

» Savor Sleep

Are you well rested? This means not being able to fall asleep in a darkened room midday. It's not normal to fall asleep if reading quietly in the afternoon or drift off at an afternoon meeting, sleep on airplanes, feel drowsy after one glass of wine, sleep when you're a passenger in a car, fall asleep watching television in the early evenings, or need caffeine and open windows to drive two hours.

Beauty sleep is not a cliché; it's a fact. When you're sleeping at night, your body enters a seemingly magical type of hibernation that allows it to repair itself. Many of the events that happen during this vital time actually cannot happen during the day and they help keep you healthy and, most of all, youthfully hydrated. Sleep medicine has come a long way in the last twenty years, and now it's a highly regarded field of study that continues to uncover surprising insights into the power of sleep in the support of health and longevity. Just about every system in the body is affected by the quality and amount of sleep you get at night. Sleep can dictate how much you eat, how fat you get, whether or not you can fight off infections, and how well you can cope with stress. The combined offenders of stress and sleep deprivation have been proven to steal precious water away from cells. This helps explain why "looking tired" typically means you're looking older and more dried out. Your skin's barrier function is compromised, and you're losing more water not only from your skin cells but from every cell in your body. There's something to be said for looking refreshed upon waking from a good night's sleep or nap.

Personal experience alone tells you what sleeplessness can do: make you look haggard and feel moody, depressed, and downright negative about everything in life. It also can encourage you to overeat, drink too much caffeine, scream at your spouse and kids, and dodge workouts and sex because you're just too tired. Sleep's profound role in our lives has also been proven over and over again in laboratory and clinical studies.[8] Among the many side effects of poor sleep habits are hypertension, confusion, memory loss, the inability to learn new information or tasks, weight gain, obesity, cardiovascular disease, and depression. How is this possible?

Sleep commands much of our well-being through our biological clocks, the natural cycle of physiological activity that changes throughout the twenty-four-hour day and is known as a circadian rhythm. This rhythm revolves around our sleep habits or, more specifically, the shifts from daytime to nighttime. A healthy day-night cycle is tethered to our normal hormonal secretion patterns, from those associated with our eating patterns to those that relate to stress, metabolism, and cellular recovery and renewal. In the morning, for example, the stress hormone cortisol should be highest and progressively decrease as the day wears on. At night, when your body senses it's dark outside, your pineal gland pumps out melatonin, which slows body functions and lowers blood pressure and, in turn, core body temperature so you're prepared to sleep. You need this hormone to achieve the deep sleep that's necessary for maintaining healthy levels of growth hormone (GH), thyroid hormone, and male and female sex hormones. If you've ever had a tough time winding down at night due to stress, you may be secreting too much cortisol, which competes with the sleep-enhancing melatonin.

Sleep is associated with the release of many hormones, some of which require you to be asleep for them to circulate. About twenty to thirty minutes after you first close your eyes and reach deep sleep, your pituitary gland, at the base of your brain, starts releasing high levels of growth hormone and will do so a few more times throughout the night in your sleep cycle. This is the most your body will secrete growth hormone in twenty-four hours. Growth hormone affects almost every cell in the body, doing so much more than just stimulating growth and cellular reproduction. It also refreshes cells and restores skin's elasticity, as well as enhances the movement of amino acids through cell membranes. It revitalizes the immune system, improves the body's usage of oxygen, lowers the risk factors for heart attack and stroke, helps prevent osteoporosis, and even aids in your ability to maintain a healthy weight. Without adequate sleep, GH won't leave the pituitary, negatively affecting your proportions of fat to muscle. Over time, low GH levels are associated with high fat and low lean muscle.

I see lots of patients who complain of uncontrollable weight gain and don't think twice about their sleep habits as they rethink their diet and exercise regimens. Yet the two digestive hormones tied to sleep habits actually control your feelings of hunger and appetite. Ghrelin (your "go eat" hormone) is secreted by the stomach when it's empty and sends a message to your brain that you need to eat. When your stomach is full, fat cells send out the other hormone—leptin— so your brain knows that you can stop eating now. One of the most exciting findings in the past decade has been how out of whack these hormones get after insufficient sleep.[9] When people are allowed just four hours of sleep a night for two nights, they experience a 20 percent drop in leptin and an increase in ghrelin. They also have a marked increase (about 24 percent) in hunger and appetite. And what do they reach for? Calorie-dense, high-carbohydrate foods like sweets and salty snacks. Sleep loss essentially deceives your body into believing it's hungry (when it's not), and it also tricks you into craving foods that can sabotage a healthy diet. What's more, because we need sleep to metabolize glucose properly, sleep loss over time can lead to diabetes. Sleep deprivation impairs the body's ability to use insulin, the hormone responsible for keeping blood sugar levels stable.

Sleep and memory also go hand in hand. By restructuring new memory representations, sleep facilitates the extraction of explicit knowledge and insightful behavior. Put simply, sleep keeps you sharp, quick-witted, creative, and able to process information in an instant. Losing as little as one and a half hours for just one night reduces daytime alertness by about one-third.

I can go on and on about the value of sleep and the casualties of not getting enough. The fact of the matter is most of us don't get the sleep we need. Sleep deprivation is epidemic. On average, we get an hour less sleep per day than we did forty years ago, and roughly two-thirds of us complain that sleep deprivation cuts into our life and well-being.

Everyone has a different sleep need. The eight-hour rule is general and not necessarily ideal for you. Most people need seven to nine hours, and chances are you know what your number is. If you feel like you're dragging after a six-hour night, then clearly you need to aim for more sleep. Think of the last time you went on vacation and slept like a baby for more hours a night than usual. *That* is probably your perfect number. Poor sleep catches up to most people, and it's not physically possible to make up a sleep loss. Despite what many people attempt to do, shifting your sleep habits on the weekends to "catch up" can sabotage a healthy circadian rhythm.

Stress and hormonal aging are the two big culprits in poor sleep, which is why it's important to establish healthy sleep hygiene—the habits that make for a restful night's sleep regardless of factors such as age, stress, and underlying medical conditions that can disrupt sleep. The goal is to minimize those factors' effects on us so we can welcome peaceful sleep. I find that women, in particular, can be more sensitive to stress in their lives and as a result, their sleep is more severely impacted. And if they turn to alcohol for relaxation at night, this in turn exacerbates the poor sleep and triggers a vicious cycle. More stress, less cellular water, heightened emotions. The key is to be mindful of the habits that have a positive or, conversely, negative impact on your sleep and aim for a good night as much as possible.

Here are eight tips for achieving sound sleep:

- Go to bed and wake up at the same time seven days a week, weekends included. Try not to fall into a cycle of burning the midnight oil on Saturday night and then sleeping until noon on Sunday. Stick to the same schedule. Your body and energy levels will love it.

- Set aside at least thirty minutes before bedtime to unwind and prepare for sleep. Avoid stimulating activities (e.g., work, cleaning, being on the computer, watching television dramas that get your adrenaline running). Try soaking in a warm bath or engaging in some light stretching. Once you're in bed, do some light reading and push any anxieties aside.

- Don't let your to-do list or worries take control. Early in the evening, say, right after dinner, write out the tasks you have yet to complete that week (not that night!) and prioritize them realistically. Add any particular worries you might have. If these notes begin to nag at you when you're trying to go to sleep, tell yourself "It's time to focus on sleep. Everything will be okay. You're tired and will have a productive day tomorrow. You're relaxed and at peace. The body needs to sleep and is ready for it."
- Reserve the bedroom for sleep only. Remove distracting electronics and gadgets, and keep it clean, cool, and dark.
- Avoid caffeine after two in the afternoon and avoid exercise at least three hours before bedtime. Watch your alcohol intake at dinner. Keep in mind that heavy foods too close to bedtime can be a digestive distraction. If you need a bedtime snack, go for simple, healthy carbs and a little fat such as a piece of toast with a spread of natural peanut butter or a handful of walnuts.
- Take better care of your body *before* going to bed than when you wake up. Give your body the tools it needs to optimize its sleep and repair itself, such as by putting a moisturizer that has antioxidants on your face and skin. Look for GABA (gamma-aminobutyric acid) in your

Aromatherapy can be very effective as a sleep aid. A great deal of scientific literature suggests that certain scents can influence mood, anxiety, immune function, and even skin health. Add some aromatherapy to your bath or keep an essential oil by your bedside. Lavender, for example, has known sleep-enhancing qualities. Other aromas linked to sensations of relaxation include rose, vanilla, and lemongrass. You can find sleep-friendly oils to dab under your nose for a calming effect. Once the fragrance of an essential oil is inhaled, nerves at the top of your nose carry it to the part of the brain that controls heart rate, memory, and hormone balance, among other things.

nighttime facial products or supplements. It acts like the body's Botox, helping your muscles to relax so they can repair themselves maximally during this important rejuvenating period. You may also want to take some extra antioxidants at nighttime, such as by eating a handful of walnuts or take an omega-3 supplement. Flooding the body with more nutrients will fuel the cellular repair shop that opens during sleep.

- Try valerian herbal tea or a chamomile blend before bedtime. Keep a sachet of lavender by your bed and take a whiff before hitting the pillow. Lavender has known sleep-inducing effects.

- Take a deep breath and release it. On your back with your eyes closed and your body stretched out, hands by your side, palms facing up, begin to tense and release your muscles starting with your head and face and working down to your toes. Breathe in deeply and slowly, telling yourself "I will fall asleep. I am going to sleep."

The whole point of sleep is to refresh the body. So you want to equip it with all the nutrients it needs to repair damage from the day. If you choose to take supplements, you may want to try taking a fatty acid supplement at bedtime that contains at least 500 milligrams of omega-3, as well as a supplement that contains antioxidants. I often recommend to patients who choose to take oral supplements for sleep that they try theanine, GABA, GLA (gamma linolenic acid), or melatonin.

» Small Shifts, Big Results

Changing the way you go about your day, from choosing what you eat to getting to bed on time, may take some time to do. I won't sugar-coat the reality: if you've been eating processed, packaged foods regularly for years and not paying any attention to getting plenty of rest, then shifting how you live won't happen overnight. And that's okay. Make it a goal to change just one thing this week in your household. If the thought of depriving yourself of the foods you currently enjoy doesn't sit well with you, simply pick up more fruits and vegetables at the market and don't change anything else. Make *additions* rather than deletions to your lifestyle at the start. You can and will wean yourself from sugary, fatty foods once you begin to incorporate nutrient-dense alternatives into your life. Your taste buds will begin to change, and you'll find yourself obsessing less over the displays at the bakery and more over the colorful array of goods in the produce section of the market. You'll start to order food differently in restaurants and be more conscious about reading labels and asking questions about how your meals are prepared.

Likewise, once you establish better bedtime habits to encourage rejuvenating sleep, you won't want to go back to earlier habits that kept you sleep deprived, moody, and chronically stressed out. Remember, this is about rebooting the body at the cellular level, which in turn helps you to turn down the volume on cultural stress and reap the rewards in a younger feeling and looking you.

CHAPTER 6

Step 3: Embrace the Power of Movement

When the ceiling gets too low, it's time to move.

Think about the last time you tried to get more active and failed. You kept up a routine for a few weeks, maybe right after New Year's, and then suddenly it was June and you didn't want to be seen in a bathing suit. You don't even remember when you fell off the wagon, but it happened. The problem for anyone trying to get active is not so much the start part as it is the *sustaining* part. At my health center, fitness and lifestyle experts help clients create a personalized, realistic plan that can be maintained. For some, that means participating in group classes at a local gym or swimming, and for others that means spending more time gardening, taking up yoga, power walking around the mall, or following a workout DVD in the family room. There is no one-size-fits-all program, so stop beating yourself up for shortcomings in the workout department. The time has come to figure out what it is that you love to do and that gets your blood running physically and psychologically. After all, movement is one of the most powerful forces against aging, including the ravages of cultural stress and depression. It's well documented, for instance, that physical activity targets the dopamine pathway and can actually be a healthy distraction when junk food is in plain view.[1]

For people already engaged in regular exercise, moving more is not such a big deal. Motivating people to be more physical when they are used to a sedentary life, however, is challenging. The secret is to exercise for pleasure. You should be driven less by exercise's health and vanity rewards than by how working out makes you *feel*. See if you can choose one activity this week (or next, if starting with your diet is enough) and plan to do more of that activity. Remember, you don't have to make a herculean effort. Go easy at the start and just get your circulation moving faster and for longer and longer periods of time. Schedule daily walks or call a friend in the morning and ask, "What can we do today?" Do jumping jacks and stretch in front of the television rather than lying on the couch. Plan a Saturday night dancing with your spouse or a group of friends. If you don't belong to a gym, ask a coworker who is a member to take you to her favorite group exercise class. You never know—you just might fall in love with it.

In fact, whether you're currently active or not, answer the following question:

If you had absolutely no obligations tomorrow, what would you do?

In my experience, the answer leads to physical activities. They may not be traditional exercises like cycling, taking an aerobics class, or using an elliptical machine, but chances are they involve activity, maybe even the outdoors. Give yourself permission to move away from traditional formats of exercise that have never worked for you in the long run, and open yourself up to exploring opportunities to get active in other, more creative ways—ways that really move you from the inside out. You'll keep coming back to them over and over again. Remember, exercise should be about pleasure, not pain (though getting sore muscles once in a while can be a very good thing; more on that below).

Giving you a specific exercise protocol is beyond the scope of this book, and if you're looking for one, then you're not getting the message. The goal is to align what *you*—just *you*—love to do with being more physical. You don't have to sweat it out at the gym or start training for a marathon. The people who boost their happy gene and achieve optimal levels of health find activities they love to do and commit to doing them more often. Simple as that.

Do what suits you, not what is expected of you.

» Not All Body Fat Is Created Equal

I am reminded every day that not all fat is created equal. I am also reminded that looks can be deceiving. A seemingly lean and skinny person can walk in and score terribly on traditional lab tests to measure health, as well as show higher-than-average body fat in a body composition analysis. I call this the Twiggy-Fat Syndrome, characterized by a low body mass index but a high fat content. People with this syndrome typically starve their cells of much-needed nutrients, forcing their bodies into starvation mode whereby they hold on tightly to fat and cannot burn energy efficiently. On the other hand, a person who carries a little extra weight but engages in physical exercise regularly will score much higher on certain lab tests used to gauge one's health status than a sedentary, unfit individual. The fitter individual has more muscle mass, which is heavier than fat pound for pound because it holds more water.

In the last decade scientists have uncovered a wealth of knowledge about the types of fat on the body. As is the case with cholesterol, good and bad types exist. Researchers have discovered an alarming difference between brown, or "good," fat and the predominant bad fat that tends to be white or yellow and collects around the waistline.[2] Brown fat, which actually has a brownish tint to it, is stored mostly around the neck and under the collarbone (so to a large extent, it's invisible). This fat encourages the body to burn calories to generate body heat and plays an important role in keeping infants warm. (Infants, we all know, do have fatty necks.) Until very recently we believed this fat was gone by adulthood or no longer active. Much to the contrary, it may have a huge role in our ability to stay lean as adults. The recent studies found that lean people have far more brown fat than overweight and obese people, especially among older folks. Unlike its bad fat counterpart, brown fat burns far more calories and generates more body heat when people are in a cooler environment. Women are more likely to have it than men, and their deposits are larger and more active.

The unhealthy fat that collects around the waistline is often referred to as visceral fat because it collects around the viscera— vital organs such as your heart, liver, and lungs. And it doesn't just sit there. Visceral fat is metabolically active, but instead of burning lots of calories, it prefers to release chemicals that affect your metabolism—negatively. Excess calories stored as body fat generate hormones that can actually cause weight *gain* while preventing the production of healthy substances that can lead to weight *loss*. We are just beginning to understand how visceral fat can change the body's chemistry and, for that matter, any attempts to lose weight and fight disease.

Visceral fat is an age maker—it wreaks havoc on our livers and has been linked to a slew of health problems including heart disease, diabetes, some forms of cancer, and a cluster of risk factors called metabolic syndrome that increases the chance of developing these diseases. It should come as no surprise that the more visceral fat you have, the lower the amount of cellular water you'll hold. I've witnessed this countless times in my practice and my lab. Remember, muscle—not fat—is the ultimate compartment for healthy water. Fatty tissue doesn't contain very much water. This explains why women are more affected by alcohol than men. If a man and a woman of the same weight but different body compositions were to drink the same amount of alcohol, the woman likely would feel its effects more strongly. Because women have a higher percentage of body fat, they cannot "dilute" consumed alcohol in the muscle mass the way a man with more muscle mass can. Her fat mass will not absorb very much alcohol, so the alcohol gets distributed in a smaller percentage of the total body mass (resulting in a higher blood alcohol content).

Visceral fat is not a problem just for overweight or obese people. You can be thin and still have visceral fat if you're not fit. While abdominal fat is usually visible, visceral fat can be hidden deep inside an outwardly thin person. The same holds true for fat that can line blood vessels, restrict blood flow, and damage the cardiovascular system.

The good news is that visceral fat isn't stuck to you forever; it responds very quickly to diet and exercise. It literally melts away when we control calories and get our bodies moving. This then paves the way to boosting cellular water. Water is the best vehicle of all for transporting fat, which makes hydration even more important. Put simply, if you want to burn fat, it must be able to be broken down and used for energy. This process, which entails a series of cellular functions, of course requires water. If the water in your blood drops below normal levels, guess what: it will pull water from your muscles to support the flow necessary in the blood. When this happens, dehydration occurs. The most fat the average person can lose in a week is roughly three pounds. If you lose more than that, it's most likely water loss.

Because visceral fat is the most dangerous kind of fat, doctors have grown more concerned about waist size than the number on the scale, which can be very deceiving. Who would you rather be: a 140-pound person with 30 percent body fat or a 145-pound person with 20 percent body fat and toned, shapely muscles? I think you'd pick the latter, and you'd look and feel a lot better, too. The secret to targeting that visceral fat? All you have to do is what I've already explained: move more. Eat more water, which will automatically help you cut calories and bathe your cells in the nutritious water that will speed up your metabolism and help burn stored fat.

You have no control over the cards that are dealt to you. But you do have control of how you play them.

» The Happy Magic of Muscle

Every year after the age of twenty-five, the average American gains one pound of body weight yet loses one-third to one-half pound of muscle. As a result, our resting metabolism decreases approximately one-half of a percent every year. So unless you downshift your caloric intake as your metabolism slows down, then you'll experience frustrating weight gain. Is this reversible? Absolutely, especially given the fact that much of this slowdown is self-perpetuated. Lifestyle changes later in life with kids, work, and hectic schedules have more and more people doing less physically.

Women have special challenges in the fat-versus-muscle department. Physiological differences are to blame, as men have ten times more testosterone than women, making it so much easier for a man to build muscle. Plus, women on average will lose muscle mass twice as fast as men the same age, and that can make a huge difference in their ability to lose or at least not gain weight. Add to that a woman's natural comparative muscle-mass-building disadvantage, and you can see why women have a harder time losing weight and keeping it off than men.

In my own studies, I've found that a person's basal metabolic rate increases as the body becomes more efficient and positively hydrated.[3] Your basal metabolic rate is the energy, measured in calories, that your body needs daily for your cells to function properly and to stay alive. It's what you burn without exerting any effort. Most women need a daily average of 1,500 to 1,800 calories; men need 1,600 to 2,200. Of course, this depends on activity levels, body size, and body type. To lose one pound of fat, you have to burn 3,500 more calories than you consume. For example, if you cut back on calories and increase your exercise so that you create a 500-calorie daily deficit, you'd burn enough extra fat to lose one pound in a week.

The math is straightforward, but the body seems to be anything but. People who go to extremes to lose weight quickly often impair their fat metabolisms by cutting too far back on calories, which forces the body into starvation mode. When this happens, the body holds tightly on to fat and burns up muscle tissue for energy—two events counterproductive to fat loss and overall health. What's more, while it's true that in theory a calorie is a calorie, the body responds differently to the source of calories. Eating a candy bar that is loaded with refined sugar and unhealthy fat will cause a spike in insulin, which triggers storage of those calories in fat cells. Eating a turkey sandwich made with whole-grain bread, bell peppers, sprouts, and avocados, on the other hand, doesn't cause a spike and requires time and an expenditure of energy to break down the proteins, healthy fats, and complex carbohydrates. The sandwich will keep your energy balanced throughout the day, support your muscles, and hydrate—rather than dehydrate—you.

People forget how valuable muscle mass is to the quality of life, longevity, and the ability to maximize metabolism. Certainly genetics and special conditions like thyroid issues can come into play when we look at weight gain and metabolic rates, but the overriding factor is muscle mass. Unlike fat, muscle is a high-maintenance tissue. It requires a lot of energy to keep it in good working order, which is why lean, more muscular people have an easier time burning calories at rest than do people with higher proportions of body fat. And it's not just about the muscle fibers that allow us to move and exercise. Think about the involuntary muscle activities that go on all the time: your heart, which itself is a muscle, pumps oxygen and nutrients to cells; muscle action pumps lymph through your lymphatic system as part of your immune system; breathing depends on muscles to deliver oxygen; and muscle activity in the skin allows us to sweat and maintain our temperature. Muscle is in constant use by the body to keep it alive and well. Muscle burns calories, whereas fat just stores them. This is why the more lean muscle you have, the faster your metabolism will be. It's the main determinant of whether your metabolism is humming at one hundred miles per hour or crawling a measly ten mph.

Although the fraction of muscle mass lost each year may seem minuscule, it actually adds up to be quite significant—translating to about a 1 to 2 percent loss of strength each year. With this loss of muscle strength, we tend to spontaneously become less active because daily activities become more difficult and exhausting to perform.

Strength Training for a Better Mood, Sleep, and a Better Body

The reason strength training gets so much attention in fitness circles is because it supports lean muscle mass and can help you increase muscle mass, strength, and bone health. While aerobic exercise improves cardiovascular fitness and burns calories (and is essential to any fitness program), it has minimal influence on muscle mass, strength, and bone health. Strength training can provide up to a 15 percent increase in the metabolic rate, which is enormously helpful for weight loss and long-term weight control. While aerobic exercise burns fat chiefly *during* exercise, strength training utilizes fat hours *after* exercise. The burn keeps going for longer than you're actually working out. Strength training also has been shown to increase bone mass, which is extremely important for women because of the increased risk of developing the brittle-bone disease osteoporosis. The muscles you engage when you lift a weight put pressure on your bones, forcing them to get stronger. In fact, loss of bone density is potentially worse than high cholesterol levels when it comes to certain types of cardio-vascular disease. Strength training provides additional benefits, too: it is an effective antidepressant and can even improve sleep quality.

Strength training can be done with free weights (e.g., barbells and dumbbells) or with universal gyms that work various parts of your body in a more controlled way. It should be done two or three times a week for about thirty minutes. Don't use weights every day. An every-other-day schedule allows your muscles to recover; try not to exercise the same muscles two days in a row.

A great way to start three days of your week, in fact, is to roll out of bed and take five minutes to stretch or perform a few bicep curls. Keep a pair of five-pound weights under your bed and complete two sets of fifteen repetitions. (With your hands at your sides each holding a weight, curl them up slowly toward your chest, then down slowly.) You'll soon begin to see more definition and feel stronger in your upper arms. Remember, the more muscle you have, the more calories you burn throughout the day—whether you are walking, vacuuming, or sleeping. This is because muscle is metabolically active. Stored fat, on the other hand, is less metabolically active, uses very little energy, and therefore burns minimal calories. Muscle equals hydration. Fat equals dehydration.

» Push Some Boundaries

As you age, it's true that your body's ability to produce an adequate supply of joint fluids, such as hyaluronic acid, diminishes, which leads to "unlubed" joints that can cause pain, inflammation, and arthritis. This then prevents a person from exercising, which further weakens joints as the condition deteriorates. The key is to stay mobile and keep your joints moving. Like the old saying goes, if you don't use it, you lose it.

It also pays to be sore once in a while after a tough workout. All improvement in any muscle function comes from stressing and recovering. Let's say one day, you work out hard enough to make your muscles burn during exercise. The burning is a sign that you are damaging your muscles. Then on the next day, your muscles feel sore because they are damaged and need time to recover. Scientists call this DOMS, or delayed onset muscle soreness.

It takes at least eight hours to feel this type of soreness. You finish a workout and feel great; then you get up the next morning and your exercised muscles feel heavy and achy. We used to think that next-day muscle soreness was caused by a buildup of lactic acid in muscles, but now we know that lactic acid has nothing to do it. Next-day muscle soreness is caused by damage to the muscle fibers themselves—due in large part to inflammation of the muscle as a result of little microscopic tears of the muscle fibers. Muscle biopsies taken on the day after hard exercise show bleeding and disruption of the filaments that hold muscle fibers together as they slide over each other during a contraction. Is this a bad thing? Far from it.

This muscle pain is a normal response to unusual exertion and is part of an adaptation process that leads to greater stamina and strength as the muscles recover and build bigger cells that can hold more nutrients and water. It's not the same as the muscle pain or fatigue you experience during exercise. This delayed pain is also very different from the acute, sudden pain of an injury such as muscle strains and sprains, which is marked by an abrupt, specific, and sudden pain that occurs during activity and often causes swelling or bruising.

So how do you know how far to push your workouts? Remember that you don't have to be training for an Olympic event to gain fitness. Next-day muscle soreness can be used as a guide to getting into and, more importantly, staying in shape. All you have to do is exercise right up to the burn, back off when your muscles really start to burn, and then pick up the pace again and exercise to the burn. This can entail simply power walking on hills. Repeat this exercise-to-the-burn-and-recover sequence until your muscles start to feel stiff, and then stop the workout. Depending on how sore your muscles feel, take the next day off or go at a very slow pace. Do not attempt to get that burning sensation again during exercise until the soreness has gone away completely. Most athletes have a very hard workout on one day, go easy for one to seven days afterward, and then have a hard workout again. World-class marathon runners run very fast only twice a week. The best weightlifters lift very heavy weights only once every two weeks. High jumpers jump for height only once a week. Shot putters throw for distance only once a week. Don't forget: exercise training is done by stressing and recovering. Stressing and recovering.

Strength in Numbers: The More You Move, the More You Burn

General dancing: 975 calories per hour*

Power walking: 600 calories per hour

Heavy or major cleaning of the house (e.g., washing the car, washing windows, cleaning the garage), with vigorous effort: 450 calories per hour

Clearing dishes from the table, washing dishes, and walking: 375 calories per hour

Watching a movie: 150 calories per hour

Numbers based on a 150-pound person

Here are other numbers you need to know. According to updated guidelines issued by the American College of Sports Medicine, engaging in moderate-intensity physical activity for 150 minutes per week (30 minutes per day, 5 days a week) may offer a great start to getting fit, but it won't necessarily prevent the march of "weight creep"—gaining weight as you get older.[4] Greater amounts of weekly physical activity—in the order of 250 minutes or more per week—is more realistic. This means 50 minutes a day, 5 days a week. Remember, though, that it doesn't have to all happen at once.

» Are You Sitting Pretty or Do You Have the Sitting Disease?

Now here's an idea few people think about every day: paying attention to posture, especially when you're sitting down at a desk hammering away at work. Posture, which is essentially how you hold yourself up and position your body, helps your muscles *stay* strong and helps your digestive system work at peak performance. It's a fact: a healthy spine supports your weight and protects your nerves and organs, enabling you to move easily throughout your day. It also protects the spinal cord and the nerves that relay messages between your brain and body.

Yoga and Pilates can help you focus on posture and improve upon it, or you can simply imagine someone pulling a string up through your body from your feet up to your head. See if you can go a day without slouching forward or leaning back.

But also beware of the sitting disease no matter how perfectly you perch yourself. You may have even read the headlines lately: sitting for prolonged periods—in spite of how fit you are—is like smoking. This means that even if you work out rigorously for an hour or more a day, you could be putting your health at risk if you're incredibly sedentary the rest of the day (e.g., commuting in your car, working at a desk, looking at screens such as a television or computer while sitting down). It turns out that just as smoking is unhealthy even if you get lots of exercise, so is sitting too much.[5] Sitting has several biological effects that negatively influence triglycerides (blood fats), high-density lipoprotein (the good cholesterol), blood sugar, resting blood pressure, and the appetite hormone leptin, which tells you when to stop eating. It can even feed depressive moods. And this is logical: when you're sitting, your circulation slows down, so those feel-good brain chemicals aren't pumping as fast. The science has been so captivating that researchers now stand by the fact that even two hours a day of exercise (which is more than the vast majority of us get) will not make up for "spending 22 hours sitting on your rear end."[6] Several of the studies have even shown that the more time people spent sitting—regardless of age, body weight, or how much they exercised—the sooner they died.[7]

So the message couldn't be clearer: we need to move and move often. Even if you do have a desk job, get up every hour for five minutes to walk around. Park at the far end of lots. Take the stairs instead of the elevator. When talking on the phone, use a wireless headset so you can walk around. Find ways to build more physical movement into your day. I know you can do this!

» Think Progress, Not Perfection

The great thing about exercise is its benefits accumulate. You don't have to go full out every day of the week for an obscene number of hours. Just twenty minutes here, a stair climb there, and ten minutes lifting weights in front of the television a few times a week can have an immediate impact. The more fit you become, the easier your exercises will feel and the more you'll want to further challenge your body. Remember, too, that as your fitness level increases, your capacity to stay hydrated will also increase naturally as you gain water-holding, fat-burning muscle mass.

> *Do what suits you, not what someone tells you to do. Period. Just as with choosing which foods you want to eat, allow the uniqueness of you to be expressed and choose what's best for you in terms of exercise. Make it your own!*

I find that patients who chart their activities each week in a journal are the most successful with maintaining a personal program and knowing when to up the ante. For example, if you don't feel a hundred percent on a Tuesday, and you look at your journal to see that you haven't moved your body in any significant way since last Wednesday, then you know that you need to schedule more activity in the coming days. It may also help you keep track of your food intake for the same reason: you'll be able to spot days when your meals aren't ideal. No one is perfect every single day, but as you chart your habits, you'll recognize progress at the same time and capture an enormous sense of satisfaction that can be very rewarding and motivating.

And sometimes *slowing down* is the secret to getting fitter. What I mean by that is if you find yourself juggling too many to-dos and losing out on quality time for yourself, you can easily watch days or even weeks go by where your good intentions fall by the wayside. Set some boundaries and tell yourself that for every week you don't fit in enough physical activity, you'll take a two- or even three-hour time-out from your normal routine to tend to your body's needs. Use that time-out to engage in a physical activity of your choice, and combine that with another activity you find stress relieving and pleasurable. Maybe it's shopping with a friend, cooking, or reading a book.

When going along the path of life, always look up.

» No Time, No Energy, No Way

If you can't fathom doing any physical exercise most days of the week between your work and family life, you're among the millions of people who struggle to schedule regular physical activity into their busy lives. Not having time and not feeling up to it are the two biggest complaints I hear. To reiterate, the secret is to find what you love to do and make that a priority in your list of tasks for the week. Don't force yourself to engage in any activities that bore you or mentally drain you. Gyms and group exercise classes are not for everyone. Also bear in mind that exercise is invigorating. As soon as you get your circulation going, those feelings of "I'm too tired" usually fade away as endorphins begin to take over. Try moving your workouts to the morning, when the day's events haven't kicked in to disrupt your schedule or wear you down. The first five minutes of exercise are the hardest, but once you get over that initial hump, the body takes over. And if you do find yourself chronically tired, then stop to ask why. Chronic exhaustion isn't a sign of health. You would do well to examine your lifestyle and priorities and attempt to reduce your stress load.

CHAPTER 7

A Seven-Day Meal Plan:
It's All about the Chocolate!

Happiness resides within.

When people claim that chocolate makes them happy, they are not bluffing. In addition to a sweetness that can trigger sensations of euphoria, chocolate has powerful chemicals that stimulate the brain's pleasure centers and can cause the brain to release feel-good hormones and substances that make you relaxed and possibly intoxicated to some degree.

But you know that you can't eat chocolate at every meal (and you'd probably get sick of it if you tried). The whole reason I titled my meal plan "It's All about the Chocolate" is to inject some fun into the task of eating and take some of the pressure out of deciding what's good versus bad to eat. Food is so stressful for a lot of people, especially those who seemingly fight the "battle of the bulge" with a battle against their food at every meal. It shouldn't be like this. Indeed, before there was medicine, there was food. But before there was food, there was chocolate! The lesson here: aim to make eating a source of not just nourishment but also joy. Don't make it complicated. And it doesn't have to be perfect.

That said, if you are ready to make a commitment to achieving a healthy body, you can make the next seven days your starting point just by focusing on your dietary protocol. And I promise it won't be difficult; remember, this is about easing up on yourself and approaching your diet in a way that's simple, easy, and pleasing. I'm all for delicious, tasty meals full of flavor and satisfaction, so that's what you're going to find here.

This nutrient blitz fills your body with everything that it needs. Luscious whole foods with all the proper nutrients will help your cells hold on to water—you'll see and feel results almost immediately. You'll find the recipe for anything marked with an asterisk (*) in appendix B.

I encourage you to limit beverages that contain caffeine, refined sugars, and alcohol during this week. Try switching to water (sparkling mineral or still) flavored with lemon, lime, or orange wedges; unsweetened fruit juices diluted with a splash of sparkling water; unsweetened iced teas; and hot herbal and green teas. If you're accustomed to drinking coffee in the morning and soda in the late morning or afternoon, see if you can reduce your intake by having just one cup of coffee with breakfast and then opt for tea rather than soda the rest of the day.

Feel free to mix and match these meal ideas; use the following outline as a guide rather than a strict regimen. Don't feel like you have to follow this meal plan to a T. If you don't like one of the ingredients listed or a meal idea, replace it! (You'll find extra recipes in appendix B; and go to www.murad.com for additional recipes and a comprehensive shopping list you can download.) Load up on the veggies, for example, but give yourself the freedom to eat them in a fashion that is as structured or unstructured as you'd like. Remember the flexible spirit of the meal plan, and you'll find it's a tasty way to better health without feeling like it's drudgery. And have fun with it! My wife and I love to make a meal by creating a stay-at-home picnic and simply grazing on our favorite vegetables, fruits, and seeds. Cut up a variety of your favorite vegetables into sticks and place them on a platter with a nice variety of citrus segments. Serve a prepared dip from your refrigerator such as hummus, black bean dip, or guacamole. And add a small bowl with a mix of your favorite seeds or nuts. It's an ideal impromptu meal that's easy to pick at while you are working on a project, reading, or sharing movie night.

After the seventh day has passed, you'll have a good sense of how a typical day of eating should go so you can then begin to make your own choices (and continue to go back to any of the ideas here that you enjoy).

Bon appétit!

» Day 1

The meal plan starts right off with one of my Stress-Free Smoothies. Every ingredient in this anti-aging power smoothie contains the key nutrients and phytochemicals to optimize the water content in the cells while also building and strengthening connective tissue. Essential amino acids to encourage the healthy formation of collagen and elastin tissue are found in the milk. Lecithin helps maintain cell membranes. The antioxidants found in the pomegranate juice, blueberries, and goji berries protect against free-radical damage to cell walls and connective tissue. Essential fatty acids found in the flaxseed lock moisture into cells. Anti-inflammatory compounds found in some of the ingredients in this smoothie help soothe skin irritation. And most importantly, the nutritional benefits of this smoothie can help increase the water content of your cells, reduce wrinkles, and increase skin elasticity.

Breakfast

Stress-Free Smoothie* of your choice

Midmorning Snack

Sliced raw vegetables (celery, cucumber, carrots, bell pepper) dipped in 2 tablespoons hummus or nut butter

Lunch

Chicken Vegetable Soup*

Veggie Sandwich on Whole-Wheat Pita* with chicken, salmon, or hummus

1 medium orange or any other fruit of your choice

Midafternoon Snack

1 whole fruit of your choice

6 raw almonds

Dinner

2 cups or more, as desired, Power Greens Salad* with 2 tablespoons Flax-Goji Golden Citrus Dressing*

4 ounces grilled salmon with tomatoes and basil

Dessert

½ cup fresh or unsweetened frozen strawberries

Tip of the Day

Flax-Goji Golden Citrus Dressing is a flavorful dressing that is great on salads and raw veggies. It provides omega-3 fatty acids (from flaxseed oil), antioxidants (from goji berries and lemon and orange juices), and B vitamins (from the nutritional yeast flakes). All these ingredients help provide your body with nutrition essentials to build healthy cells.

» Day 2

Breakfast

½ medium grapefruit (optional: sprinkle with stevia or drizzle with agave nectar)

1 cup low-fat Greek-style yogurt sprinkled with chia seeds or flaxseeds

Midmorning Snack

1 whole fruit of your choice

6 raw almonds

Lunch

1 cup cooked whole-wheat pasta topped with 1 cup steamed mixed vegetables (broccoli and cauliflower florets, carrot and zucchini slices) and 2 ounces cooked skinless white meat chicken (cut into cubes), or ½ cup baked and cubed tofu, covered with ½ cup marinara sauce

Midafternoon Snack

2 tablespoons dried goji berries or raisins

4 raw walnuts

Dinner

4 ounces grilled wild fish of your choice with lemon and dill

½ cup steamed brown rice

Roasted Greens*

Dessert

Fresh fruit platter (a wide variety of colorful fruits) with ½ cup Greek-style or soy yogurt

---

Tip of the Day

There has been a lot of controversy regarding the popular sugar substitutes on the market. For those who can't do without their regular dose of sweetness, I recommend a sweet herb called stevia. Stevia has been used worldwide for more than four hundred years without any reported side effects. Interestingly, in South America, where the herb is plentiful, the leaves have been used for centuries as a natural medicine for type 2 diabetes. It's extremely popular in Japan, where it's been used for decades. Stevia has a sweetness that is two hundred to three hundred times greater than sugar. A new product called Truvia has emerged on the market, and this is a stevia-based sweetener that you can now find in grocery stores. Another natural sweetener to try is agave nectar, which is produced from the live agave plant and comes in liquid form. You can find agave nectar at most grocery stores. Drizzle it over low-fat Greek-style yogurt sprinkled with a handful of dried goji berries and crushed walnuts in the morning and you've got yourself a luscious breakfast.

And if you have a sweet tooth and are in need of a serious but healthy sugar fix, overripe bananas, yams, and sweet potatoes can do the trick with or without the agave or stevia added.

» Day 3

Breakfast

½ cup old-fashioned oatmeal with cinnamon and raisins or dried goji berries with fat-free milk or soy milk
1 medium orange

Midmorning Snack

1 cup or more, as desired, raw vegetables of your choice topped with Dr. Murad's Favorite Salsa*

Lunch

2 cups or more, as desired, tossed green salad with 2 tablespoons dressing of your choice
2 cups Hearty Moroccan Chicken*

If you buy prepared salad dressing, opt for brands that are all-natural. Avoid dressings that are high in sugar and artificial ingredients such as high fructose corn syrup, modified cornstarch, and monosodium glutamate. You do not need to opt for fat-free varieties, but be careful about portions. Use a measuring spoon to drizzle a single serving of dressing over a salad.

And when preparing a mixed green salad, try to incorporate as much variety of green leafy vegetables as you can. Be adventurous—try new types of greens and lettuces in your salads. Experiment. Try bitter greens—they are important health supporters. As a general rule, the darker the greens, the better the nutrition. The more variety you can use, the more increased nutrition and the more new flavors you can enjoy.

Midafternoon Snack

Stress-Free Smoothie* of your choice

Dinner

1 cup steamed broccoli sprinkled with grated parmesan

4 ounces grilled fish with lemon juice or 4 ounces grilled vegetarian soy "chicken"

½ cup brown rice pilaf

Dessert

Apple "Pie" with Berry Sauce*

Tip of the Day

Oatmeal is one of the best whole grains to include in a heart-healthy diet. It includes soluble fiber to help lower cholesterol, and this fiber also is beneficial in keeping blood sugar under control. Oats are also a natural source of antioxidants.

Oranges and other citrus fruits are high in the antioxidants vitamin C and bioflavonoids. These antioxidants prevent oxidation and damage to our cells by free radicals. Whole oranges (but not orange juice) are also a good source of fiber.

In the Pitcher of Health, nonfat and low-fat yogurt is included as a protein food. Yogurt also is a good source of calcium and riboflavin. It contains friendly bacteria that can replenish the friendly bacteria in our intestines after the supply dwindles. In North America, the two most common friendly bacteria strains used to make yogurt are *Streptococcus thermophilus* and *Lactobacillus bulgaricus*. These two types of friendly bacteria change the milk's sugar (called lactose) into lactic acid, which is responsible for yogurt's tangy taste. If you don't eat dairy products, soy yogurt is widely available and is an excellent alternative.

Broccoli is high in vitamin A (beta carotene) and vitamin C, two important antioxidants to protect our cells from damage. The vitamin A and various phytochemicals, such as isothiocyanates, indoles, and bioflavonoids, in broccoli may help prevent cancer. Broccoli is also a good source of calcium.

» Day 4

Remember, the meal plan is not a low-carb diet plan. In fact, it includes plenty of healthy carbs that provide the body the nutrients and energy it needs for optimal health. In this diet plan, we emphasize eating only whole grains, not the refined processed grains that most Americans eat too much of and that turn quickly into sugar. Whole grains are complex carbohydrates and provide important fiber as well as essential nutrients like B vitamins.

Breakfast

The Doctor's Veggie Scramble*
1 slice whole-grain toast with 100 percent whole fruit jam or spread

Midmorning Snack

1 cup red or purple grapes
1 ounce cheese of your choice

Lunch

2 cups or more, as desired, tossed green salad with 2 tablespoons dressing of your choice
Deli sandwich of your choice on whole-grain bread

Midafternoon Snack

1 cup or more, as desired, raw vegetables of your choice with optional salad dressing as a dip
6 raw almonds

Dinner

2 cups White Bean and Cherry Tomato Salad*

Steamed Vegetables with Marinara*

Avocado Lime Parsley Chicken*

Dessert

1 serving dark chocolate (at least 70 percent cocoa)

Tip of the Day

While generally I recommend eating most of your fruits and vegetables fresh and uncooked, you can cook your vegetables in ways to minimize their nutrient loss during preparation. One of the best and most nutritional ways to cook vegetables is to steam them by placing them on a rack or in a basket above boiling water. The food should not touch the water because nutrients can be lost in the water. Lightly steamed vegetables are excellent as they retain many of the important nutrients found in their uncooked state.

Microwaving vegetables is a quick and nutritional way to cook vegetables with little or no water. You can also minimize the fat in this type of food preparation. Be sure not to overcook your vegetables when using the microwave—cook them for only short periods of time.

Stir-frying with small amounts of olive or canola oil and water or vegetable broth is another nutritious way to prepare your vegetables. When stir-frying, be sure to cook the vegetables until just tender and use as little oil or liquid as possible to retain nutrients.

» Day 5

Breakfast

2 eggs any style with a whole-wheat English muffin

1 medium orange or other fruit of your choice

Midmorning Snack

1 cup or more, as desired, raw vegetables of your choice with optional salad dressing as a dip

Lunch

Red Cabbage Salad*

Roasted turkey sandwich on whole-grain bread with Dijon mustard, tomatoes, and avocado

1 medium apple

Midafternoon Snack

½ or 1 sliced raw bell pepper dipped in 2 tablespoons hummus

Dinner

Grilled chicken breast with sauce of your choice

1 cup steamed brown rice

Roasted Greens*

Dessert

Banana Mousse*

Tip of the Day

Getting your essential amino acids from healthy protein foods is important for the formation of collagen and elastin tissue. The Pitcher of Health includes protein selections that are best for building healthy cells by providing the body with essential amino acids. Fish and skinless white-meat poultry are better choices of protein. Of fish, salmon and black cod are ideal choices because they are rich sources of omega-3 fatty acids, the type of fat essential to having healthy, hydrated cells. Studies also suggest that omega-3 fatty acids play a role in protecting against cardiovascular disease and enhancing brain function. And don't forget about the incredible, edible egg. Many people forgo eating eggs because of cholesterol concerns; however, eggs provide nutrients that act as precursors to women's hormones and can play an important part in staving off hormonal aging.

They also provide vitamins B and A, as well as iron. Just as dietary fat is not the same as body fat, dietary cholesterol is not the same as blood cholesterol. In other words, just because you eat eggs doesn't mean you'll automatically raise your cholesterol. A lot more is going on at the biological level. When possible, it's best to look for eggs with boosted vitamin E levels.

Try to get protein from plant sources as well. By doing so, you are getting your amino acids from the original source of amino acids—plants. Eating vegetable protein foods as opposed to animal sources of protein has many health benefits. Vegetable proteins contain no cholesterol or saturated fat and in many cases also provide a good source of dietary fiber.

» Day 6

Breakfast
½ grapefruit
Bowl of low-sugar, whole-grain cereal with low-fat milk or almond milk, topped with a handful of fresh blueberries

Midmorning Snack
Stress-Free Smoothie* of your choice

Lunch
Asparagus-Orange Salad*
Avocado-vegetable sandwich on whole-grain bread

Avocados are known for their high fat content; however, they contain healthy monounsaturated fat and contain no cholesterol. So they're a healthy choice that not only enhances your overall condition but makes your skin glow. Avocados contain lutein, a phytochemical with important antioxidant properties.

Midafternoon Snack
6 raw walnuts
Carrot or celery sticks, as many as desired

Dinner

Tomato slices, as many as desired, with vinaigrette dressing
5-ounce grilled salmon steak or grilled vegetarian soy burger patty
Swiss Chard with Caramelized Onions and Goji Berries*
Whole-wheat roll lightly brushed with olive oil

Dessert

¼ cup ricotta cheese sprinkled with cinnamon and topped with
1 cup blueberries

Tip of the Day

In the Pitcher of Health we list only whole grains. Refined-grain foods and products are not part of the meal plan. This is because when you refine grains, you take away their nutritional value. Whole grains include wheat, corn, rye, oats, barley, quinoa, and spelt—when these grains are eaten in their "whole" form. Whole grains even include popcorn! Eating whole grains has been shown to reduce the risks of heart disease, stroke, cancer, diabetes, and obesity. These nutrient-rich gems contain important antioxidants, B vitamins, and fiber, protein, minerals, and healthy fats. Eating whole grains (and avoiding refined grains) is an important part of a healthy diet.

» Day 7

Breakfast

Stress-Free Smoothie* of your choice
½ cup old-fashioned oatmeal with cinnamon and fat-free milk or soy milk
½ medium cantaloupe or 1 cup cubed cantaloupe

Midmorning Snack

1 serving organic, wholesome trail mix (skip the sugary kinds with candy or milk chocolate)

Lunch

White Bean and Cherry Tomato Salad*

1 cup Gazpacho Soup*

1 medium apple

Midafternoon Snack

1 cup or more, as desired, raw vegetables of your choice with optional salad dressing as a dip

1 cup fat-free, 1 percent, or soy milk or ½ cup low-fat cottage cheese

Dinner

2 cups or more, as desired, tossed green salad with 2 tablespoons dressing of your choice

Asian Stir-Fry Vegetables with Chicken or Tofu*

½ cup cooked brown rice

Dessert

½ cup fresh or frozen unsweetened blueberries

Tip of the Day

Low in saturated fat and rich in heart-healthy monounsaturated fats and flavor, olive oil is an excellent vegetable oil to have in your kitchen. Extra-virgin olive oil is considered the finest olive oil. Extra-virgin olive oil is made, without heat or solvents, from the first pressing of the olives. It is the most flavorful of the different types of olive oil, and most importantly, extra-virgin olive oil contains the highest amount of healthy polyphenol antioxidants of all olive oils. I recommend using extra-virgin olive oil when preparing foods.

After following the diet and menu plan for seven days or more, you should begin to feel improvements in your health and well-being, although it'll probably take longer to see the results in your physical appearance. Don't worry: this first week accomplished a lot, especially if you began to incorporate the ideas outlined in the three steps.

This menu plan is not simply just another diet that you follow for only a specified time. It is a nutritional lifestyle guide you should continue to follow the rest of your life. This is vital to keep your body, right from the cellular level, functioning at its optimal level. The meals and recipes in this meal plan are examples of the types of foods and diet needed to achieve optimal health and well-being. I encourage you to continue on this nutritional path of healthy eating, which is critical to your ongoing success in following my program. By doing so, you will reap the benefits of a long and healthy, happy life.

Remember, happiness resides within. Now go cultivate it!

365 Statements to Say to Yourself throughout a Year

1. Why have a bad day when you can have a good day?
2. Before there was medicine, there was food.
3. Aging is a fact of life. Looking your age is not.
4. Healthy skin is a reflection of overall wellness.
5. Healthy, hydrated cells are the key to ageless skin and a healthy body.
6. We are each born with a unique commodity called life. It is stressed by the environment, and it is up to us to make the best of it.
7. When you come to a wall in the road, life is telling you to make a turn.
8. You have no control over the cards that are dealt to you. But you do have control of making the best of them.
9. Magic happens only when you create your own.
10. Be comfortable with who you are.
11. Be imperfect; live longer.
12. Learn from the vagaries of life.
13. Even in disaster, look for the good.
14. Smile daily; frown infrequently.
15. Look out of the box for solutions to your problems.

16. Happiness resides within.
17. Before there was surgery, there was Inclusive Health.
18. Don't let failure spoil your success.
19. Ignore the naysayers from without and, more importantly, those from within. Allow yourself to achieve your maximum potential.
20. Have only big, flexible dreams with no limits—so your potential will have no limits.
21. Be too big for your britches.
22. Remember the healing power of pride.
23. Lead yourself.
24. Stay in touch with your passion.
25. Don't let the vagaries lead to vacancies.
26. Stay ahead of the curve, even though it is a lonely journey.
27. Allow spontaneity in your life.
28. Equal parts of vegetables and vegging out keep the doctor away.
29. The largest explosion starts with a few grains of sand.
30. Eighty percent of health resides in the brain.
31. Eat your water—don't drink it.
32. Be friends with your passion.
33. If it's not personal, don't take it personally.
34. Turn the rest of your life into the best of your life.
35. Isolation can be a self-imposed prison.
36. When the ceiling gets too low, it's time to move.
37. Take pleasure in every minor success.
38. The best is yet to come; you just have to let it enter.
39. Explore your hidden opportunities.
40. Find your hidden potential.
41. Water loss is the final common pathway to all aging and disease.
42. Make trailblazing a way of life.

43. Be more efficient; reduce waist.
44. Rewrite and reframe the negatives in your life.
45. Reduce Internet isolation—sleep better.
46. Let others help you.
47. Splurge often.
48. In order to learn, ask yourself before asking others.
49. Life is good, bad, and indifferent—focus on the good.
50. Feel that you are about to improve and you will.
51. Evolve quickly to reach your goal.
52. Learn from your disability.
53. Live young.
54. When going through the path of life, always look up.
55. Many shortcuts turn into long cuts.
56. Die late, not old.
57. Before there was a revolution, there was an evolution.
58. Resolution requires concentration.
59. Be consistent with your message, but be sure it's flexible enough to be transformed.
60. Increase simplicity in your life.
61. Reduce complexity in your life.
62. Be thrilled with who you are.
63. Make your house your home.
64. Listen to yourself so you can pay attention to your needs.
65. Unify a diverse message.
66. Reduce the number of your daily decisions.
67. When making a difficult decision, solitude is a necessary element.
68. Transformation can happen in twelve weeks.
69. Take each day as an opportunity to grow.
70. Share your love.
71. Inclusive Health reduces waist.
72. The Water Principle is the unifying method of reducing

aging, disease, and wrinkles.

73. Progress starts when you cut the umbilical cord.
74. Success comes by cutting your own umbilical cord and allowing freedom.
75. Medicine is imperfect; you have to look at it inclusively.
76. Surround yourself with happiness.
77. Bear hugs keep the doctor away.
78. Enjoy intimacy.
79. Remember the healing power of love.
80. Find elements of health from around the world.
81. The healing power of water.
82. Take others along the path with you.
83. Treat yourself as royalty.
84. The ultimate cellular need is water.
85. Opportunities abound; keep your eyes open for them.
86. Expect less; be happy.
87. Make additions rather than deletions to your lifestyle.
88. Detoxify your body with plants.
89. Improve your immunity with plants.
90. Think positive; detoxify your brain.
91. Start a revolution.
92. Reality, not rhetoric.
93. If you can't find it, you may be looking for the wrong thing.
94. When you fall down, get up quickly.
95. Be someone special.
96. Find your direction and focus on it.
97. Heal yourself; reduce isolation.
98. Opportunity comes to those who ask.
99. Perfectionism leads to pessimism.
100. There is a difference between having fun and being happy.
101. Be brave enough to make difficult decisions.

102. When you become the most important person to yourself, your accomplishments will amaze you.
103. Make Inclusive Health your destiny.
104. Celebrate the privilege of making your own decisions.
105. Enjoy the privilege of doing purposeful work.
106. Be stable during times of instability.
107. Failure is the path to success.
108. Don't be so hard on yourself.
109. Beware of creating your own stress.
110. Embrace Inclusive Health—the no-diet weight loss plan.
111. Water is necessary for cell function.
112. If you haven't failed, you haven't succeeded.
113. Look for what you can't find; it may actually be in front of your eyes.
114. Don't wait to do your bucket list.
115. It's not just the science but the art of health.
116. Competency trumps genius.
117. Cultural stress equals attention deficit hyperactivity disorder.
118. Cultural stress equals dependency and addiction.
119. Attitude trumps intelligence.
120. Learn from your mistakes; don't project them on others.
121. If you put what you are worrying about in perspective, it's probably no big deal.
122. When you are smitten, it is important to maintain your own persona.
123. Don't become used and abused.
124. Lifestyle can modify genes.
125. Embellish your genes.
126. Improve your genes.
127. Make your mark, but allow the canvas of life to direct you.
128. Allow happiness to enter.

129. Replenish your passion.
130. Restore youth.
131. You are valuable; don't sell yourself short.
132. When you learn to be imperfect, your life will be more perfect.
133. Technology can turn the impossible into the possible.
134. Create a competitive advantage.
135. Your best is better than the competition.
136. Your competitive advantage is doing your best.
137. Failure comes when you don't try.
138. Success comes when you try.
139. Fear of failure leads to failure.
140. Success comes when you don't fear failure.
141. Success comes when you accept the possibility of failure.
142. Go for it, no matter how unattainable it may seem.
143. It may just be your turn.
144. Believe you are good enough for_____.
145. Look for random events that can change your life.
146. Return to your youth.
147. Begin to know exactly what you want.
148. Think of yourself as royal, not poor.
149. Give yourself permission to be successful.
150. Give yourself permission to have your own opinion.
151. Give yourself permission to be happy.
152. Give yourself permission to make changes in your life when appropriate.
153. In order to reach your potential, you must risk failure.
154. Opportunity changes luck.
155. Open yourself for an opportunity to be lucky.
156. Don't measure yourself against unattainable goals.
157. To be happy, don't measure yourself against others.
158. Don't set yourself up for unrealistic expectations.

159. Survive despite being damaged.
160. If permitted, failure leads to success.
161. Before there was medicine, there was food; before there was food, there was chocolate.
162. Give yourself permission to say no.
163. You are worthy of_____.
164. Expose your accomplishments to others without fear of rejection.
165. Accept the potential for the unexpected.
166. Accommodate, but don't let your life be turned upside down.
167. Accommodate, but maintain your power.
168. Accommodate, but realize what you are doing.
169. Accommodate, but expect to be recognized for it.
170. Accommodate, but don't be disconnected.
171. Become yourself.
172. Be heard.
173. Be thankful.
174. Be interested.
175. Project happiness.
176. Project self-confidence.
177. Project loving and caring.
178. Transitions are imperfect road maps to the future. It is up to you to make the best of them.
179. Make the best of transitions in your life.
180. Make transitions into an opportunity for positive changes.
181. Maintain your power during transitions in your life.
182. Think of transition as an opportunity.
183. Allow transitions to have a powerful impact on you.
184. During times of darkness, look for illusions of light and warmth.
185. Find beauty everywhere.

186. Color darkness with bright colors.
187. Your accomplishments will be enhanced only when you expose them to others without fear of rejection.
188. Live in a healthy physical and emotional environment to reach your full potential.
189. Choose the best environment for you.
190. Find a complete environment that breeds success and happiness for you.
191. If it is no big deal, don't make a big deal about it.
192. As you progress, maintain your soul.
193. Give yourself permission to be healthy.
194. Expect health.
195. Think healthy.
196. Expect to be healthy.
197. Encourage healing.
198. Let health enter.
199. Choose health.
200. When you are comfortable with yourself, your accomplishments will amaze you.
201. Be brave enough to expose yourself to your harshest critic.
202. Be comfortable in yourself to free others.
203. Have intentions to improve.
204. Your harshest critics are really very critical of themselves—not you.
205. Follow your path despite what others think.
206. Be yourself; don't emulate.
207. Develop a basic recipe for your healthy life to allow it to be modified over time.
208. Understand the source of healthy nutrition.
209. Find education wherever it resides.
210. You can catch more fish with a net than a hook.

211. Remember to wear your crown.
212. Begin to know when something is enough.
213. Focus on your ultimate goals and not the steps getting there.
214. Don't blame your second-grade teacher for your failures.
215. When life looks bleak, look for a window for change.
216. The road to success runs through managing change.
217. Make sure you can buy gas before you buy a car.
218. Life always throws curve balls—you need to learn to hit them out of the park.
219. Happiness means finding beauty every day.
220. Think inspiration before perspiration.
221. Wait for the big fish that loves you by making yourself better while you wait.
222. The message can always be messaged depending on the messenger's point of view.
223. If you want to be miserable every day, you will find something that went wrong even if 99 percent went right.
224. Give yourself permission to_____.
225. Accept the possibility that your expectations won't be met.
226. Think of it as an opportunity when your expectations are not met.
227. Be interested so you can become interesting.
228. When you have intentions to_____, it is more likely to happen.
229. Understand the real reason for your decisions.
230. When medical therapy exposes your body to a new environment, take it as an opportunity for a positive change.
231. To address life's ever-increasing fast-paced changes, you need to be flexible.
232. Don't focus on the minutiae in life.
233. Make your journey without a destination.

234. Happiness does not require luxury.
235. Think of your life as a vacation.
236. Removing barnacles from your skin begins to remove the barnacles from your brain, which will allow positive thoughts to enter your mind and body.
237. Without healing, there is no health.
238. When making a decision, details matter.
239. Give yourself permission to be generous.
240. Give yourself an opportunity to have a transformation.
241. Wherever you are on life's journey, there is an opportunity for positive change.
242. Become a champion in your own league.
243. Sometimes one key can open many doors.
244. Be happy even when your expectations are not met.
245. Believe you are good enough to take care of yourself.
246. Become free to_____.
247. Your life's story in the end is how you have lived it. Make it sweet, happy, and healthy.
248. Learn from yourself.
249. Allow the unique you to blossom.
250. Develop your unique power.
251. Your life's story is based on your developing it.
252. You have the ability to develop your life story.
253. You have it in your power to_____.
254. Allow yourself to take a chance.
255. Eat your success.
256. Develop the world future yesterday.
257. Invent the future today.
258. Water-rich foods are the best diet plan.
259. Let others help you by taking the first step.
260. Free those you love.
261. Don't deal with what you could have done. Deal with what

you are going to do.

262. Become a champion in your own division.
263. The right key can open many doors.
264. Become free to be yourself.
265. Just be.
266. Embrace the little things you do; they may become really big things.
267. Honor yourself.
268. Try laughter when you are in pain.
269. See sunshine in gray skies.
270. Many different problems have the same solution.
271. Your harshest critic may have become you yourself.
272. Let yourself speak.
273. Be prepared for your first success—it sometimes comes accidently.
274. Real truth is probably 70 percent of the real truth. Thirty percent depends on individual interpretation—it is up to you to learn the real truth.
275. Understand the real truth of your life.
276. Learn who you really are.
277. Find your calling.
278. Learn from others, but establish your own journey.
279. Champion your own decisions.
280. Eat your medicine.
281. It's not the stress; it is how you respond to it.
282. Be careful of advice—it may come from a person's insecurities.
283. If you keep banging your head against the wall, you will have a headache no matter how many pain pills you take.
284. Inhibitions increase with age; stay young.
285. The least of us may become the best of us.
286. Heal yourself; allow the unique you to blossom.

287. Handouts may turn into holdouts.
288. Handouts may reduce your potential.
289. Handouts don't always pay out.
290. Be comfortable with who you are, not who you could have been or should have been.
291. Realistic expectations can go beyond what you are theoretically entitled to.
292. You never know until you try.
293. Delete negative self-talk.
294. Positive self-talk encourages a positive outcome.
295. Youth building is the path to positive self-talk.
296. Replace cultural stress plus negative self-talk with a positive attitude.
297. Youth building neutralizes cultural stress.
298. Reduce stress—increase total body hydration.
299. Give yourself permission to be loved.
300. Give yourself permission to have a passion.
301. Developing your passion is a major step in the journey to happiness.
302. Make an appointment with yourself.
303. Forgive yourself.
304. Handouts may not be helpful.
305. Focus on what you can do, not what you can't do.
306. Allow your disability to transform your abilities.
307. Learn by watching without judging.
308. Don't let others embarrass you.
309. Don't judge others when they embarrass themselves.
310. Reconcile yourself to the truth, and then make the best of it.
311. Don't allow your disability to brand you.
312. Powerful lessons taught can have a powerful impact on the teacher as well as the student.

313. Learn from your mistakes.
314. Many of our life lessons emanate from mistakes we have made.
315. Real change happens only when you create your own.
316. You need to become yourself; do what fits you—such as diet, job, hobby, clothes—not what you think others expect of you.
317. Your skin is connected to your heart. Make your heart happy and your skin will become more beautiful.
318. You will be most happy when your loved ones are happy.
319. Be happy when you see happiness in others.
320. Eat to hydrate your brain, allowing happiness to enter.
321. Make your heart happy and your skin will glow.
322. Do what fits you, not what others expect of you.
323. You were your real self before you were two; to really progress, you need to become yourself.
324. Open yourself to the opportunity to be loved.
325. When you love others, you will become loved.
326. Cherish your loved ones.
327. Open your heart to love.
328. Forgive yourself first before you forgive others; then both of you can heal.
329. Help yourself and others by not critically judging so that all are given permission and freedom to learn from mistakes.
330. When you are happy, your loved ones will be happy.
331. When you make your own journey, you release others to do the same.
332. Consider the cost benefit before you get angry.
333. Become authentic.
334. Give yourself permission to be the real you—the toddler in you.

335. The right answer is not always the right answer.
336. Give yourself permission to make decisions by learning from yourself.
337. Giving without limits may in the end make you an enabler.
338. By asking for help, you give yourself and others permission to be loved.
339. If you can think it, it could happen.
340. Create new opportunities without fear of failure.
341. Medicine works best when the patient is accepting of it.
342. Take care of the most important person in your life—you.
343. Instead of leading a horse to water, give him permission to take his own path so he will be more likely to drink.
344. Become important to yourself.
345. Unlock your hidden potential.
346. Allow the unique you to blossom.
347. Real paradise exists only in your mind, not a physical location.
348. When you make yourself your chief competitor, you succeed by doing your best.
349. Art is medicine.
350. The best health tip is to smile.
351. Increasing simplicity allows your ultimate goals to enter.
352. Increasing gene expression requires the science plus the art of medicine.
353. Spontaneity leads to a more fulfilling life.
354. Learn from the toddler in you.
355. Be thrilled with who you are, not what you could have been, not who you should have been.
356. Learn from others, but understand them through your own prism to be able to go to the next level.
357. Don't just think out of the box; think as if there were no

box.

358. When choosing a doctor, go to one that treats patients' illnesses rather than illnesses' patients.
359. Be brave enough to expose yourself to your harshest critic without fear of rejection.
360. Become younger—be more inquisitive; don't take things for granted.
361. Make sure you make the best of your days as time and life fly by.
362. "Healing" has more letters than "health"; therefore it must be more important.
363. Don't blame yourself for other people's problems.
364. You are responsible only for your own problems.
365. Don't feel guilty for being yourself.

Recipes

» The Stress-Free Smoothies

Cellular Water Smoothie

- ½ cup pomegranate juice (unsweetened)
- ½ cup soy, low-fat, or nonfat milk
- ½ cup blueberries (fresh or unsweetened frozen)
- 1 tablespoon lecithin granules
- 1 tablespoon ground flaxseed
- 2 tablespoons dried goji berries
- 3 to 4 ice cubes or crushed ice (optional)
   Stevia extract or agave nectar (optional) to taste

Combine all ingredients in a blender and blend until smooth.

Tropical Protein Smoothie

- 1 cup pineapple juice
- ½ banana
- 1 scoop soy protein isolate powder
   Crushed ice

Combine all ingredients in a blender and blend until smooth.

Tip: For more energy add 2 tablespoons dried goji berries.

Veggie Antioxidant Smoothie

   ¾ cup fresh carrot juice

   ¼ cup fresh natural unfiltered apple juice

   2 dark green lettuce leaves

   2 spinach leaves

   ¼ cup chopped fresh broccoli

   2 sprigs parsley

   ½ teaspoon diced ginger root

Combine all ingredients in a blender and liquefy.

Wake-Up Shake (Smoothie)

   1 cup soy or almond milk

   ½ cup pineapple

   ½ cup kale

   1 banana

      Ice, if desired

Combine all ingredients in a blender and blend until smooth.

The Doctor's Veggie Scramble

   1 to 2 cups raw vegetables (try scooping from a bag of mixed, precut veggies)

   1 tablespoon lentils (cooked)

   1 to 2 eggs

      Canola oil or cooking spray

Add lentils to one or two scrambled raw eggs in a bowl.

Drizzle olive oil in a skillet or use an olive oil cooking spray to coat the bottom. Cook raw vegetables until slightly soft.

Pour egg mixture on top of veggies, combine all ingredients, and cook until egg is done.

Chicken Vegetable Soup

Makes 6 servings

- 2 cups vegetable broth
- 1 cup fresh or frozen corn kernels
- 1 celery stalk, diced
- 1 small carrot, diced
- 1 small onion, diced
- 1 cup cooked skinless, boneless chicken breast, diced or shredded
- ½ cup diced tomatoes
- 2 tablespoons finely chopped fresh parsley
- Salt and pepper to taste

In a saucepan, combine the vegetable broth, corn, celery, carrot, and onion. Bring to a boil.

Reduce the heat, cover, and simmer for 25–30 minutes or until the vegetables are tender.

Stir in the chicken, tomatoes, parsley, and salt and pepper. Heat thoroughly.

Vegetarian Split Pea with Barley Soup

Makes 6 servings

- 1 cup split peas, rinsed and drained
- 2 carrots, diced
- 2 stalks celery, diced
- 1 medium onion, minced
- 6 cups water or vegetable broth
- ¼ cup barley, rinsed and drained
- 1 bay leaf
- ¾ teaspoon reduced-sodium sea salt
- ⅛ teaspoon white pepper

⅛ teaspoon dried parsley

⅛ teaspoon dried thyme

1 clove garlic, minced

½ tablespoon lemon juice

1 tablespoon extra-virgin olive oil

Chopped scallions, for garnish

In a large soup pot, combine the split peas, carrots, celery, onions, and water or broth. Bring to a boil.

Stir in the barley, bay leaf, sea salt, pepper, parsley, thyme, garlic, lemon juice, and olive oil. Reduce the heat and simmer, partly covered, for 1½–2 hours. Occasionally stir as needed. Add additional salt and pepper to taste if desired.

When the soup has become thick, turn off the heat. Cover and let it sit for 15 minutes. Discard the bay leaf. Stir. Garnish with chopped scallions.

Gazpacho Soup

Makes three 1-cup servings

2 cups low-sodium V8 juice

¼ cup chopped raw turnip

½ cup peeled, seeded, chopped cucumber (about ½ medium cucumber)

¼ cup chopped celery

¼ cup chopped yellow pepper

¼ cup chopped sweet onion

¼ cup chopped carrots

Freshly ground black pepper to taste

Put juice and vegetables into a blender and process very briefly. Season with freshly ground black pepper.

Asparagus Orange Salad

Makes 4 servings

- 1 pound thin asparagus
- 1½ cups watercress
- ½ small red onion, very thinly sliced
- 1 orange cut into 12 segments
- 1 tablespoon fresh orange juice
- 1 teaspoon orange zest
- 1 teaspoon stevia
- 1 tablespoon red wine vinegar
- 2 teaspoons sunflower seeds
- 2 tablespoons extra-virgin olive oil
- Pepper to taste

Blanch the asparagus for 2 minutes in boiling water. Rinse under cold water to cool. Place in a serving dish and combine with watercress, onion, and orange segments. Combine the orange juice, orange zest, stevia, red wine vinegar, and sunflower seeds in a small bowl, whisk in the oil; and drizzle dressing over salad. Season with freshly ground black pepper.

Kale Salad with Almonds and Avocado

Makes 4 servings

- 1 bunch lacinato (dinosaur) kale (or other tender, baby kale), washed, center ribs removed, and leaves roughly chopped
- 2 oranges
- 3 tablespoons olive oil
- ½ avocado, diced
- 2 tablespoons sliced toasted almonds
- Freshly ground black pepper
- Reduced-sodium sea salt to taste

For dressing: Combine the juice of one orange with the olive oil, reduced-sodium sea salt, and pepper. Mix until very well combined. Set aside.

To assemble salad: Peel the second orange and separate the sections, peeling off the white pith as best as possible. Chop orange sections roughly and place in a bowl with the chopped kale leaves, diced avocado, and almonds. Drizzle about half the dressing over the salad and toss well to coat. Season with freshly ground black pepper before serving.

Salad will keep well for a couple of days in a covered container in the fridge. Dressing will keep well in a sealed jar for about a week.

White Bean and Cherry Tomato Salad

Makes 4 servings

    1 15-ounce can cannellini beans, rinsed and drained
    2½ cups halved grape or cherry tomatoes
    ⅔ cup diced red onion
    ¼ cup chopped fresh dill
    ¼ cup extra-virgin olive oil
    3 tablespoons fresh lemon juice
    1 tablespoon balsamic vinegar
    2 garlic cloves, pressed
       Pepper to taste

Toss all ingredients in a large bowl. Season with freshly ground black pepper. Marinate at room temperature 1 hour.

Red Cabbage Salad

Makes 2 cups

    ½ medium red cabbage chopped
    1 green Granny Smith or pippin apple, sliced into fingers and then chopped
    1 cup fresh lemon juice
       Pinch of reduced-sodium sea salt (optional)

As it sits in the refrigerator this mixture becomes a beautiful bright pink color.

It's a great side dish on its own or can be mixed with another salad like the Power Greens Salad (see below).

Power Greens Salad

Always keep a Power Greens Salad base and healthy add-ins in the refrigerator. New power greens mixes available in many markets include great greens such as baby kale, baby chard, and baby spinach. These blends make a terrific healthy base for you to customize and create your own special salads. If you cannot find a prepared power greens mix in your local market, experiment with what you can find—you may need to start with bagged spinach or kale and mix it with one bag of cabbage prepared for coleslaw. When your power greens lose their peak freshness for salads, lightly steam them for side dishes; sauté them with poultry, fish, or egg dishes; or make a vegetable soup or smoothie with them. Be creative with vegetables and you will love the results!

Use your imagination and have fun adding in a selection of favorite healthy foods that you have on hand to the power base.

My favorite Power Greens Salad add-ins include whole grains, nuts, seeds, fruits, tofu, tempeh, seafood, fish, poultry or lean meat, cucumbers, fennel, baby bok choy, broccoli, the entire cabbage family, celery, turnips, all colors of peppers, fresh herbs, carrots, the radish family, fresh sprouted veggies and grains, sugar snap peas, chayote squash, cauliflower, avocado, artichoke hearts, hearts of palm, shredded beets, sun-dried tomatoes, fresh tomatoes, fresh chopped ginger, lentils, quinoa, garbanzo beans, kidney beans, black beans, flaxseeds, pumpkin seeds, sunflower seeds, sesame seeds, walnuts, slivered almonds, pine nuts, pomegranate seeds, blueberries, blackberries, goji berries, citrus segments, sliced pears, and sliced apples.

» Dressings

Flax-Goji Golden Citrus Dressing

Makes 2 cups

- ½ cup flaxseed oil
- ½ cup water
- ¼ cup fresh lemon juice
- ¼ cup fresh orange juice
- ¼ cup dried goji berries (or dried cranberries)
- 3 tablespoons nutritional yeast flakes
- 2 tablespoons Bragg Liquid Aminos or tamari soy sauce
- 1 tablespoon apple cider vinegar

Combine all ingredients in a blender and blend until smooth. Store in a well-sealed jar in the refrigerator for up to two weeks.

Olive Oil and Lemon Juice Dressing

Makes about ¼ cup, enough for 4 salads

- 3 tablespoons extra-virgin olive oil
- 1 tablespoon fresh lemon juice
- ½ small clove garlic, finely minced
- 1 teaspoon reduced-sodium sea salt

In a small bowl, mix all ingredients vigorously with a wire whisk.

Olive Oil and Red Wine Vinegar Dressing

Makes ¾ cup

- 4 tablespoons extra-virgin olive oil
- ½ cup apple cider vinegar
- 3 cloves fresh garlic, minced
- ⅛ teaspoon dried oregano
- ⅛ teaspoon dried thyme

Place all ingredients in a glass container with a lid. Cover and shake vigorously.

Balsamic Vinaigrette Dressing

Makes ¾ cup

- ½ cup extra-virgin olive oil
- ¼ cup good balsamic vinegar
-    Chopped garlic (about four cloves)
-    Chopped shallots (about 1 tablespoon)
- 1 tablespoon Dijon mustard
- ½ tablespoon light soy sauce
- ½ tablespoon agave nectar
-    Rosemary (fresh or dried) to taste
-    Fresh lemon juice to taste
-    Pepper to taste

Combine all ingredients together *except* for the oil. Then drizzle the oil slowly into the mixture as you whisk it.

Veggie Sandwich on Whole-Wheat Pita

You can add 3 ounces of cooked, cubed chicken breast or cooked, cubed salmon to the sandwich.

-    Tomatoes, ½-inch diced
-    Red onion, ½-inch diced
-    Black olives, chopped
-    Whole-wheat pita, cut in half to form two pockets
- 2 lettuce leaves
- ¼ cup hummus

Mix together the tomato, onion, and olives.

Place a lettuce leaf in each pocket. Stuff the pockets with the vegetables and hummus.

Steamed Vegetables with Marinara

Makes 4 servings

- 2 cups broccoli florets
- 2 cups cauliflower florets
- 2 medium carrots, diagonally cut
- 1 cup string beans, diagonally cut
- 2 medium zucchini, cut into ¼-inch rounds
- 2 medium green, red, or yellow bell peppers (or a combination), cut into 1-inch strips
- 1½ cups low-fat marinara sauce, heated

Over a pot of boiling water, lightly steam the vegetables in a steamer basket until they are cooked but still crunchy.

Arrange the vegetables on a platter. Top with low-fat marinara sauce.

Asian Stir-Fry Vegetables with Chicken or Tofu

Makes 4 servings

Vegetable Stir-Fry

- 1½ tablespoons soy sauce or Bragg Liquid Aminos
- ¼ cup vegetable broth or water
- 2 teaspoons canola oil
- 2 teaspoons minced garlic
- 1 teaspoon minced fresh ginger
- 1 large carrot, diagonally sliced in small strips
- 1 cup celery, diagonally sliced in small pieces
- 1 cup snow peas, stems and strings removed
- 2 medium red bell peppers, cut into 1-inch strips
- 1 cup fresh mushrooms
- 1 cup scallions, diagonally sliced (including green tops)

Combine the soy sauce or Bragg Liquid Aminos, vegetable broth or water, and canola oil.

Heat a nonstick wok or skillet over high heat and add the soy sauce mixture. Add the garlic, ginger, carrot, celery, snow peas, peppers, mushrooms, and scallions. Stir constantly while cooking over high heat for about 2 minutes. Add small amounts of additional water if needed. The vegetables should be tender and crisp.

Add prepared chicken or tofu (see recipes below), if desired, and blend thoroughly. Cook until desired temperature and texture. Serve with brown rice.

Prepared with Chicken

   2 teaspoons tamari soy sauce or Bragg Liquid Aminos
   2 teaspoons rice vinegar
   ½ teaspoon minced fresh ginger
   ½ teaspoon minced garlic
   2 tablespoons vegetable broth
   4 cooked boneless, skinless chicken breast halves, fat trimmed and cut into ½-inch strips

In a bowl, combine the tamari or Bragg Liquid Aminos, vinegar, ginger, garlic, and vegetable broth.

Add the chicken pieces and toss together. Cover the bowl and refrigerate for about ½ hour.

Add the chicken mixture to the wok and stir-fry.

Prepared with Tofu

   ¼ cup tamari soy sauce or Bragg Liquid Aminos
   ½ teaspoon minced fresh ginger
   ½ teaspoon minced garlic
   1 package (14 ounces) firm tofu, well drained and cut into ½-inch cubes

Preheat the oven to 350°F. In a bowl, whisk together the soy sauce or Bragg Liquid Aminos, ginger, and garlic.

Add the tofu and gently stir to coat each cube.

Spread the tofu on an oiled baking sheet and bake for a few minutes, until the tofu is hot and golden on the outside. You may need to move the cubes around on the baking sheet with a spatula so they heat evenly while baking.

Steamed Tofu

½ cup firm tofu, cut into ½-inch cubes

4 tablespoons tamari soy sauce or Bragg Liquid Aminos

¼ teaspoon minced ginger

In a steamer, lightly steam the cubed tofu for 5 minutes.

Flavor with a mixture of soy sauce and minced ginger. Or you can use any fat-free flavorful sauce.

Dr. Murad's Favorite Chili

Makes 5 servings

1 tablespoon canola or grape seed oil

1 cup chopped onions

1 medium red bell pepper, cored, seeded, and cut into ½-inch cubes

1 tablespoon chili powder (to taste)

1 teaspoon red pepper flakes (to taste)

½ teaspoon turmeric

1 teaspoon minced fresh ginger

¼ teaspoon curry powder

½ teaspoon dried oregano

1 rounded tablespoon fresh chopped garlic (to your taste)

1 pound lean chicken or lean turkey

1 15-ounce can kidney beans (or other beans), drained

1 14.5-ounce can Mexican or Italian stewed tomatoes, coarsely chopped

Salt-free herbal seasoning blend (to taste)

Heat the oil in a Dutch oven over medium heat; sauté onions, bell pepper, chili powder, and all spices; then add garlic. Stir until the vegetables are softened and beginning to brown. Increase the heat to medium high, add the poultry, breaking up the chunks with a spoon, and cook until it is just beginning to brown.

Add beans, tomato puree, stewed tomatoes, and salt-free herbal seasoning blend. Bring mixture to almost a boil, and then reduce heat to a simmer. Cover and cook, stirring occasionally so the chili does not stick. If it becomes too thick, add ¼ cup of water. Cook until flavors blend and adjust the seasonings to taste.

Chicken and Black Bean Burrito

- 4 ounces chicken
- ½ cup cooked black beans
- ¼ cup steamed fresh or frozen corn kernels, broccoli florets, and ½-inch diced carrots or other favorite vegetables
- 1 low-fat whole-wheat tortilla
- ½ cup Tomato Salsa (recipe below)

Cut chicken into cubes and pan-fry using a light cooking spray until cooked. Combine the beans and vegetables. Place the mixture on the tortilla. Add the chicken. Wrap the tortilla to form a burrito. Top with Tomato Salsa.

Beans, Greens, and Pasta

Makes 4 servings

- 6 ounces whole-wheat penne pasta
- 2 tablespoons of extra-virgin olive oil
- 1 onion, chopped
- 3 cloves garlic, chopped
- 1 bunch kale, center ribs removed, chopped
- 1 cup low-sodium vegetable broth
- 1 15-ounce can low-sodium cannellini beans (or other small white bean), drained and rinsed

1 teaspoon cayenne pepper

Freshly ground black pepper to taste

Cook penne as directed. Set aside. Heat olive oil in a large skillet. Add onions and gently sauté until caramelized (about 20 minutes). Add garlic and simmer an additional 2 minutes. Add chopped kale and cook until wilted. Add vegetable broth and cannellini beans. Cook for 5 minutes. Add pasta. Season with cayenne pepper and freshly ground black pepper.

Tilapia with Artichoke and Lemon

Makes 4 servings

1 pound fresh tilapia fillets

4 teaspoons Dijon mustard

½ cup artichokes (in a jar or frozen), chopped

2 tablespoons lemon juice

⅓ cup white wine

Preheat oven to 350°F. Lay the tilapia in a single layer in a baking dish. Spread with mustard. Add ½ cup cut-up artichokes. Pour lemon juice and wine over dish and bake for 20 minutes.

Vegetable Turkey Burger

Makes 4 servings

1–2 tablespoons extra-virgin olive oil

1 onion, diced

1 bell pepper, diced

16 ounces 100 percent breast meat turkey

1 small zucchini, grated

1 egg, beaten

1 tablespoon cayenne pepper

2 tablespoons Dijon mustard

½ cup bread crumbs

Gently sauté onion in about 1 tablespoon olive oil until golden brown, about 20 minutes. Add bell pepper and simmer until tender. Add to large bowl and mix with remaining ingredients. Shape into 4-ounce patties. (The shaped burgers can be frozen.) Cook in oiled pan on medium heat until cooked through. Top with fresh onion, tomato, avocado, lettuce, or vegetables of your choice.

Papaya-Stuffed Chicken

Makes 6 servings

    2 chicken breasts
    1 onion, finely chopped
    1 tablespoon extra-virgin olive oil
    1 egg
    2 tablespoons soy mayonnaise
    ½ teaspoon Dijon mustard
    1 tablespoon dried dill or ¼ cup chopped fresh dill
    1 teaspoon dried ginger
    3 celery stalks, chopped
    ½ cup artichokes (in a jar packed in water), chopped
    ¼ cup chopped walnuts
    ¼ cup dried goji berries
    ¼ cup plus 1 tablespoon whole-wheat bread crumbs
    1 large ripe papaya

Grill chicken and cut into 2-inch pieces. Sauté onion in olive oil. Whisk egg in a separate bowl. Add mayonnaise, mustard, dill, and ginger. In a large mixing bowl, mix chicken, sautéed onions, chopped celery and artichokes, walnuts, goji berries, and ¼ cup of bread crumbs. Combine with egg-mayonnaise mixture. Cut papaya in half, remove seeds, and cut a small slice from the bottom of each half (so papaya can sit flat). Spoon chicken mixture into the hollow of each side of the papaya. Sprinkle 1 tablespoon of bread crumbs over chicken mixture. Bake at 325°F for 35 minutes.

Hearty Moroccan Chicken

Makes 4 servings

   2 tablespoons extra-virgin olive oil
   4 chicken leg quarters, skinned
   1 medium onion, cut in chunks
   4 cloves garlic, minced
   1 tablespoon minced fresh ginger
   2 carrots, peeled and cut in chunks
   1 cup no-salt-added canned chickpeas, rinsed and drained
   ½ cup golden raisins
   2 sticks cinnamon
  1½ teaspoons cumin
   ½ teaspoon turmeric
   2 cups low-sodium chicken broth
   3 cups water
   2 zucchinis, cut in chunks

Put olive oil into large, nonstick skillet and place over high heat. Add chicken and cook about 10 minutes, turning to brown on all sides. Stir in onion, garlic, ginger, carrots, potatoes, chickpeas, raisins, cinnamon, cumin, turmeric, chicken broth, and water. Bring to a simmer, reduce heat, and cook about 20 minutes. Stir in zucchini and cook an additional 10 minutes. Remove cinnamon sticks. A one-dish meal!

Avocado Lime Parsley Chicken

Makes 2 servings

   1 ripe avocado
   6 ounces cooked chicken, diced
   4 tablespoons chopped walnuts
   1 cup grapes, quartered
   ¼ cup chopped fresh parsley
      Pepper to taste

Mash avocado in a medium-sized bowl. Combine with remaining ingredients. Season with freshly ground black pepper.

Cinnamon Spice Salmon

Makes 4 servings

- ½ teaspoon cayenne pepper
- 1 tablespoon cinnamon
- 1 teaspoon ground ginger
- 1 pound salmon fillet

Combine spices. Place salmon fillet on foil in a baking pan, skin side down. Sprinkle spices on surface of salmon. Bake at 350°F for 20 minutes. For more kick, increase cayenne pepper to 1 teaspoon.

Rice and Red Lentil Pilaf

Makes 4 servings

- 2 tablespoons olive oil
- 1 large onion, chopped
- 3 cloves garlic, chopped
- 1 tablespoon garam masala
- 1 cup brown basmati rice
- 1 cup red lentils
- 3 cups low-sodium vegetable stock

Heat oil in saucepan. Add onion, garlic, and garam masala. Cook over low heat for 10 minutes until onions are soft. Stir in the rice and lentils and cook for 2 minutes. Add the stock and stir well. Slowly bring to a boil, reduce heat, cover, and simmer for 20 minutes or until the broth has been absorbed. Gently fluff the rice with a fork.

Quinoa Tabouleh

Makes 5 servings

- 1¾ cups water

1 cup uncooked quinoa

½ cup coarsely chopped seeded tomato

½ cup chopped fresh mint or parsley

¼ cup raisins

¼ cup chopped cucumber

¼ cup fresh lemon juice

2 tablespoons chopped green onions

1 tablespoon extra-virgin olive oil

2 teaspoons minced fresh onion

¼ teaspoon salt-free herbal seasoning blend

¼ teaspoon freshly ground black pepper

Combine water and quinoa in a medium saucepan; bring to a boil. Cover, reduce heat, and simmer 20 minutes or until liquid is absorbed. Remove from heat; fluff with a fork. Stir in tomato and remaining ingredients. Cover; let stand 1 hour. Season with freshly ground black pepper. Serve chilled or at room temperature.

Tomato Salsa

2 cups chopped tomatoes

⅓ cup chopped onions

1 4-ounce can chopped green chilies

¼ cup finely chopped fresh cilantro

2 tablespoons fresh lime or lemon juice

¼ teaspoon reduced-sodium sea salt

Hot sauce to taste

Place all ingredients in a large mixing bowl and blend thoroughly.

Mango Salsa

1 ripe mango, diced

1 tomato, diced

1 small white onion, diced

¼ cup chopped fresh cilantro

1 jalapeno, diced

2 teaspoons extra-virgin olive oil

1 tablespoon fresh lime juice

Combine all ingredients in a mixing bowl. This salsa tastes better if it marinates for a couple of hours in the refrigerator.

Dr. Murad's Favorite Salsa

1 medium avocado, chopped into medium-sized chunks

½ bunch cilantro, chopped fine

3 to 4 tomatoes, chopped into small cubes

1 tablespoon fresh lemon juice (about 1 lemon)

1 teaspoon extra-virgin olive oil

Pinch reduced-sodium sea salt to taste

Mix above in a medium-sized bowl. Can be used as a dip or a salad dressing. Adding garlic aioli creates another light version of the salad dressing. This salsa can be made with limes.

Hummus

Makes four ½-cup servings

2 cups cooked or canned garbanzo beans (chickpeas)

⅓ cup fresh lemon juice

¼ cup tahini

2 cloves garlic

2 teaspoons extra-virgin olive oil

1 teaspoon salt (reduced-sodium sea salt)

½ teaspoon onion powder

¼ cup water

Fresh parsley, chopped (for garnish)

Combine all ingredients in a blender and blend until very smooth. Add additional water if necessary. Garnish with chopped parsley. Sprinkle paprika and sumac on top.

Roasted Greens

Makes 4–6 servings

- 1–2 pounds Brussels sprouts
- 1 large head broccoli
- 1 tablespoon chopped fresh thyme leaves or 1 teaspoon dried
- 1 tablespoon chopped fresh oregano leaves or 1 teaspoon dried
- 1 teaspoon garlic powder
- ½ teaspoon kosher salt
- ¼ teaspoon freshly ground black pepper
- ¼ cup extra-virgin olive oil
- ½ cup reduced balsamic vinegar

Heat oven to 425°F.

In a bowl, combine Brussels sprouts and broccoli florets. Drizzle extra-virgin olive oil over the veggies to lightly coat them. Add the thyme, oregano, garlic powder, salt, and pepper. Pour contents of the bowl onto a roasting pan and cook for 20 minutes. Shake the contents and cook for another 20 to 25 minutes until the veggies are browned. Drizzle vinegar over the top while hot and serve.

Roasted Carrots

Peel some thin carrots. Preheat oven to 425°F. Spray a roasting pan with olive oil cooking spray. Place carrots—or any vegetable of your choice—on the pan and drizzle with 2 tablespoons olive oil. Shake the pan so all carrots are coated with oil. Bake for 15 minutes. Shake pan again and cook an additional 15 minutes until carrots are tender and golden brown.

Swiss Chard with Caramelized Onions and Goji Berries

Makes 4 servings

- 2 tablespoons chopped walnuts
- 1 tablespoon extra-virgin olive oil
- 1 large sweet onion, coarsely chopped
- 1 large bunch Swiss chard, rinsed well
- ¼ cup dried goji berries
- 2 tablespoons balsamic vinegar
- Freshly ground black pepper to taste

In a large skillet or Dutch oven, toast the walnuts over low heat, stirring frequently, until golden brown, about 2 minutes. Transfer to a plate and set aside to cool. In the same pan, heat the oil over medium-low heat. Add the onions and cook, stirring occasionally, until golden brown and very soft, 9 to 12 minutes. Meanwhile, cut the center ribs from the Swiss chard, cut into 2-inch strips, and place in a saucepan. Cover with water and simmer until tender. Drain water.

Tear the Swiss chard leaves into 2-inch pieces. Add Swiss chard leaves and vinegar to the caramelized onions and cook, stirring occasionally, until the leaves are wilted, about 5 minutes. Add tender ribs. Season with freshly ground black pepper. Transfer to a serving dish and top with goji berries.

Apple "Pie" with Berry Sauce

- Extra-virgin olive oil spray
- 3 apples, peeled and sliced
- Berry sauce (recipe below)

Lightly spray pie pan with olive oil spray. Arrange apple slices on pie pan. Broil (not too near to heat) until golden, about 10 minutes. Pour ½ cup berry sauce over the apples. Store the remaining pureed berries for tomorrow's breakfast smoothie. Serve warm.

Berry Sauce

> 1 10-ounce package frozen berries (blueberries or raspberries or mixed berries), thawed
>
> 1 tablespoon lemon juice

Puree mixed berries in food processor. Add lemon juice.

Banana Mousse

> 1 bunch of soft bananas
>
> 1 tablespoon of organic honey
>
> 1 tablespoon of almond butter
>
> Pumpkin seeds

Blend bananas, honey, and almond butter together until smooth. Spoon mixture into champagne flutes and add pumpkin seeds on top. Chill until ready to serve.

Notes

Chapter 1

1. For access to my studies on cultural stress, go to http://www
   .murad.com and click on Conquering Cultural Stress.

2. Ibid.

Chapter 2

1. A. Steptoe et al., "Enjoyment of Life and Declining Physical
   Function at Older Ages: A Longitudinal Cohort Study," *Canadian
   Medical Association Journal* 186, no. 4 (March 4, 2014): E150–E156.

2. Daniel Kahneman and Angus Deaton, "High Income Improves
   Evaluation of Life but Not Emotional Well-Being," *Proceedings of the
   National Academy of Sciences.* (September 7, 2010), doi:10.1073
   /pnas.1011492107. See also Shigehiro Oishi et al., "Concepts
   of Happiness across Time and Cultures," http://www-bcf.usc.
   edu/~jessegra/papers/OGKG.inpress.HappinessConcepts.PSPB.pdf.

3. Jon Clifton, "Latin Americans Most Positive in the World," Gallup
   World, December 19, 2012, http://www.gallup.com/poll/159254
   /latin-americans-positive-world.aspx#1.

4. See the OECD Better Life Index, http://www.oecdbetterlifeindex.
   org/.

5. Alexander Weiss, Timothy C. Bates, and Michelle Luciano,
   "Happiness Is a Personal(ity) Thing: The Genetics of Personality and
   Well-Being in a Representative Sample," *Psychological Science* 19, no.

3 (March 2008): 205–210. Also see Michael Mendelsohn, "Positive Psychology: The Science of Happiness," ABC News, January 11, 2008, http://abcnews.go.com/Health/story?id=4115033&page=1&singlePage=true.

6. To view the results of my genetic study, go to http://www.murad.com.

7. R. N. Butler et al., "New Model of Health Promotion and Disease Prevention for the 21st Century," *British Medical Journal* 377, no. 7662 (2008), doi:10.1136/bmj.a399.

8. Centers for Medicare and Medicaid Services, *Chronic Conditions among Medicare Beneficiaries, Chartbook: 2012 Edition* (Baltimore: CMS, 2012), http://www.cms.gov/Research-Statistics-Data-and-Systems/Statistics-Trends-and-Reports/Chronic-Conditions/Downloads/2012Chartbook.pdf.

9. Butler et al., "New Model of Health Promotion."

10. C. A. Jackson and G. D. Mishra, "Depression and Risk of Stroke in Midaged Women: A Prospective Longitudinal Study," *Stroke* 44, no. 6 (2013): 1555–1560, doi:10.1161/STROKEAHA.113.001147.

11. M. Tanasescu et al., "Physical Activity in Relation to Cardiovascular Disease and Total Mortality among Men with Type 2 Diabetes," *Circulation* 107 (2003): 2435–2439. See also F. B. Hu et al., "Walking Compared with Vigorous Physical Activity and Risk of Type 2 Diabetes in Women: A Prospective Study," *Journal of the American Medical Association* 282, no. 15 (1999): 1433–1439. For a comprehensive, well-cited review of preventable actions on diabetes, see Harvard School of Public Health, "Simple Steps to Preventing Diabetes," http://www.hsph.harvard.edu/nutritionsource/preventing-diabetes-full-story/.

Chapter 3

1. See "Our Story," Blue Zones, http://www.bluezones.com/about/.

2. M. Jackowska et al., "Short Sleep Duration Is Associated with Shorter Telomere Length in Healthy Men: Findings from the Whitehall II Cohort Study," *PLoS ONE* 7, no. 10 (2012): e47292, doi:10.1371/journal.pone.0047292.

3. Hans Selye, "A Syndrome Produced by Diverse Nocuous Agents," *Nature* 138, 32-32 (July 4, 1936) doi:10.1038/138032a0.

4. *Online Etymology Dictionary*, s.v. "stress," www.etymonline.com /index.php?term=stress.

5. To access a database of average annual hours actually worked per worker in various countries, go to the Organization for Economic Co-Operation and Development's website at http://stats.oecd.org.

6. P. H. Ryan et al., "Is It Traffic Type, Volume, or Distance? Wheezing in Infants Living Near Truck and Bus Traffic," *Journal of Allergy and Clinical Immunology* 116, no. 2 (2005): 279–284.

7. See "Stress at Work," Centers for Disease Control and Prevention, www.cdc.gov/niosh/topics/stress/.

8. See "Mental Health Basics," Centers for Disease Control and Prevention, www.cdc.gov/mentalhealth/basics.htm. Also check out the following: C. J. L. Murray and A. D. Lopez, *The Global Burden of Disease: A Comprehensive Assessment of Mortality and Disability from Diseases, Injuries and Risk Factors in 1990 and Projected to 2020* (Boston: Harvard School of Public Health, 1996).

9. See American Psychological Association, *Stress in America: Missing the Health Care Connection* (Washington, DC: APA, February 7, 2013, http://www.apa.org/news/press/releases/stress/2012/full-report.pdf.

10. Kate Karelina et al., "Social Isolation Alters Neuroinflammatory Response to Stroke," *Proceedings of the National Academy of Sciences* 106, no. 14 (April 7, 2009): 5895–5900.

11. R. L. O'Sullivan, G. Upper, and E. A. Lerner, "The Neuro-Immuno-Cutaneous-Endocrine Network: Relationship of Mind and Skin," *Archives of Dermatology* 134, no. 11 (1998): 1431–1435, doi:10.1001/archderm.134.11.1431.

12. Sobia Kauser et al., "Modulation of the Human Hair Follicle Pigmentary Unit by Corticotropin-releasing Hormone and Urocortin Peptides," *FASEB Journal* 20, no. 7 (May 2006): 882–895.

Chapter 4

1. Anna Magee, "Trying to Be Perfect Could Be Ruining Your Health: It Can Trigger Heart Disease, IBS and Insomnia—and Some Experts Say It Could Even Be as Bad for You as Smoking," *Daily Mail*, April 14, 2014, http://www.dailymail.co.uk/health/article-2604621 /Trying-perfect-ruining-health-It-trigger-heart-disease-IBS-

insomnia-experts-say-bad-smoking.html#ixzz30JZkVrMm.

2. For a list of studies detailing the effects of perfectionism on health, see Dr. Danielle Molnar's work at Brock University's Department of Psychology (www.brocku.ca).

3. Lynn C. Giles et al., "Effect of Social Networks on 10 Year Survival in Very Old Australians: The Australian Longitudinal Study of Aging," *Journal of Epidemiology & Community Health* 59 (2005): 574–579, doi:10.1136/jech.2004.025429.

4. William Harms, "AAAS 2014: Loneliness Is a Major Health Risk for Older Adults," *UChicago News*, February 16, 2014.

5. Nicholas A. Christakis and James H. Fowler, "The Spread of Obesity in a Large Social Network over 32 Years," *New England Journal of Medicine* 357, no. 4 (July 25, 2007): 370–379.

6. M. Maria Glymour et al., "Social Ties and Cognitive Recovery after Stroke: Does Social Integration Promote Cognitive Resilience?" *Neuroepidemiology* 31, no. 1 (2008): 10–20.

7. A. M. Grool et al., "Structural MRI Correlates of Apathy Symptoms in Older Persons without Dementia: AGES-Reykjavik Study," *Neurology* 82, no. 18 (May 6, 2014): 1628–1635, doi:10.1212 /WNL.0000000000000378.

8. P. A. Balaji, Smitha R. Varne, and Syed Sadat Ali, "Physiological Effects of Yogic Practices and Transcendental Meditation in Health and Disease," *North American Journal of Medical Sciences* 4, no. 10 (2012): 442–448.

9. H. Lavretsky et al., "A Pilot Study of Yogic Meditation for Family Dementia Caregivers with Depressive Symptoms: Effects on Mental Health, Cognition, and Telomerase Activity," *International Journal of Geriatric Psychiatry* 28, no. 1 (2013): 57–65, doi:10.1002/gps.3790.

10. To access a library of studies about the power of massage over stress, visit the American Massage Therapy Association at http://www.amtamassage.org. Also check out the Touch Research Institute's site at the University of Miami School of Medicine, http://www6.miami.edu/touch-research/About.html.

11. Ibid.

12. Ibid.

Chapter 5

1. Aaron E. Carroll and Rachel C. Vreeman, *Don't Swallow Your Gum! Myths, Half-Truths, and Outright Lies about Your Body and Health* (New York: St. Martin's Griffin, 2009).

2. Gregory McNamee, "Eight Glasses (of Water) a Day: The Origins of a Nutritional Adage," Encyclopedia Britannica Blog, September 12, 2012, http://www.britannica.com/blogs/2012/09/glasses-water-day-origins-nutritional-adage/.

3. J. N. Hall et al., "Global Variability in Fruit and Vegetable Consumption," *American Journal of Preventive Medicine* 36, no. 5 (2009): 402.

4. Centers for Disease Control and Prevention *State Indicator Report on Fruits and Vegetables 2013* (Atlanta: CDC, 2013), http://www.cdc.gov/nutrition/downloads/State-Indicator-Report-Fruits-Vegetables-2013.pdf. Also see Steven Reinberg, "Most Americans Still Not Eating Enough Fruits, Veggies," *US News & World Report*, September 9, 2010, http://health.usnews.com/health-news/diet-fitness/diet/articles/2010/09/09/most-americans-still-not-eating-enough-fruits-veggies.

5. Melinda Beck and Amy Schatz, "Americans' Eating Habits Take a Healthier Turn, Study Finds," *Wall Street Journal*, January 16, 2014.

6. David G. Blanchflower, Andrew J. Oswald, and Sarah Stewart-Brown, "Is Psychological Well-Being Linked to the Consumption of Fruit and Vegetables?" National Bureau of Economic Research, NBER Working Paper No. 18469, October 2012, http://www.nber.org/papers/w18469.

7. C. Bernard Gesch et al., "Influence of Supplementary Vitamins, Minerals and Essential Fatty Acids on the Antisocial Behaviour of Young Adult Prisoners," *British Journal of Psychiatry* 181 (2002): 22–28, doi:10.1192/bjp.181.1.22.

8. To access up-to-date news and studies about sleep, go to the National Sleep Foundation's website at http://www.sleepfoundation.org.

9. Ibid.

Chapter 6

1. N. R. Lenard and H. R. Berthoud, "Central and Peripheral Regulation of Food Intake and Physical Activity: Pathways and Genes," *Obesity* 16, suppl. 3: S11–S22, doi:10.1038/oby.2008.511.

2. Qiong A. Wang et al., "Tracking Adipogenesis during White Adipose Tissue Development, Expansion and Regeneration," *Nature Medicine* (2013), doi:10.1038/nm.3324. For more about the different types of fat, see the work of Dr. Bruce Spiegelman: http://cellbio.med.harvard.edu/people/faculty/spiegelman.

3. Visit http://www.murad.com and click on Conquering Cultural Stress.

4. "ACSM, AHA Support Federal Physical Activity Guidelines," American College of Sports Medicine, http://www.acsm.org/about-acsm/media-room/acsm-in-the-news/2011/08/01/acsm-aha-support-federal-physical-activity-guidelines.

5. A. V. Patel et al., "Leisure Time Spent Sitting in Relation to Total Mortality in a Prospective Cohort of US Adults," *American Journal of Epidemiology* 172, no. 4 (2010): 419–429, doi:10.1093/aje/kwq155.

6. D. W. Dunstan et al., "Too Much Sitting—a Health Hazard," *Diabetes Research and Clinical Practice* 97, no. 3 (2012): 368–376, doi:10.1016/j.diabres.2012.05.020.

7. P. T. Katzmarzyk et al., "Sitting Time and Mortality from All Causes, Cardiovascular Disease, and Cancer," *Medicine and Science in Sports and Exercise* 41, no. 5 (2009): 998–1005, doi:10.1249/MSS.0b013e3181930355.

Index

biological process of aging, 42–43
Blue Zones, 60–61
body categories, Hippocrates's, 31
body fat, 121–124
body systems, homeostasis of, 47
bone density, 126
brain
    dopamine pathway, 98
    nourishing your, 105–106
    shrinkage of, 85
breast cancer, 34
breathing, 86
Britain, gross domestic happiness
        (GDH) measure in, 18–19
British Medical Journal, 42, 43
brown fat, 121–122
Buddhist principles, 19

C

calories, 73, 122, 124–125, 126,
        129
*Canadian Medical Association
        Journal,* 16
cancer, 34, 87, 96, 106, 107, 122,
        142, 146
capsaicin, 107
carbohydrates, 98, 114
    complex, 95, 101, 125, 142
    refined, 101
cardiovascular system, 46
Carroll, Aaron E., 92–93
cayenne pepper, 107
CDC (Centers for Disease Control),
        94
cells
    appearance of healthy and
        unhealthy, 26
    damage to, 29
    description, 36–37
    renewal ability of, 41
    vulnerability during aging of, 31
    water loss from, 76
cellular aging, 86
cellular turnover, 46–47, 72
cellular water, 24. *See also* water/
        water intake
    in body fat, 48–49

building lean muscle for sup-
        porting, 49
    contentment and, 51
    effects of protocols for increas-
        ing, 25–26
    health related to content of, 25
    problems of loss of, 24–25
Cellular Water Smoothie, 165
Centers for Disease Control (CDC),
        94
changes, making small, 117–118
chemical transmitters, 74
Chicken and Black Bean Burrito,
        177
Chicken Vegetable Soup, 167
children/infants
    cultural stress in, 70–71
    effects of stress on, 68, 69
    stress in, 76
chili, 107
cholesterol, 144–145
    HDL and LDL, 105, 130
chronic diseases, 32, 43
chronic stress, 65, 66
Cinnamon Spice Salmon, 181
circadian rhythm, 112–113, 115
Circle of Life, 52
citrus fruits, 141
coffee, 108
cognitive elements of happiness,
        21, 22
cognitive stress, 67
collagen, 38, 46–47, 101, 144
communication, lack of, 60
comorbidity, 42–43
complex carbohydrates, 95
connecting to others, 84–85
    disconnecting, 85–86
    planning time for, 88–89
connective tissues, 31, 37, 46–47
contentment, cellular water content
        and, 51
corticotropin-releasing hormone
        (CRH), 72, 74
cortisol, 49, 72–73
    effects on sleep of, 113
creativity, 14–15

About the Author

Howard Murad, M.D., FAAD, is a board-certified dermatologist, trained pharmacist, Associate Clinical Professor of Medicine (Dermatology) at the Geffen School of Medicine, UCLA, and founder of Murad Skincare, Inc. Fondly known as the Father of Internal Skincare, he has changed how the world sees skincare through his pioneering research and clinical studies into Cultural Stress and The Science of Cellular Water™, one of the world's most comprehensive approaches to understanding health and aging. Dr. Murad's Inclusive Health philosophy sets him apart from other dermatologists and general practitioners, as it emphasizes that skin is not only the body's largest organ but is connected to, and reflective of, the health of all systems in the body. Holding eighteen patents, Dr. Murad has been named an "Industry Visionary" by the International SPA Association and a "Beauty Genius" by *Elle* magazine and recently received the first Aesthetic Visionary Award for Lifetime Achievement. He is the author of five previous books that share practical lifestyle choices as the path to looking and feeling as healthy, happy, and beautiful as possible.